Acknowledgments

I owe special thanks and gratitude to so many people for their support of RopeSport and this book that it's difficult to know where to start.

At the very top of my thank-you list is undoubtedly Mara Tyler. Mara's official title was Project Manager, but that in no way adequately describes her involvement in helping to bring this book to fruition. Her organizational skills, creativity, intelligence, and work ethic throughout this process were truly amazing. Mara's many contributions to this book cannot be emphasized enough.

Special thanks to my editor, Christel Winkler (no relation), for her skill and insight during this process. Additional thanks to all the people at my publisher, John Wiley & Sons, who believed in this project and gave me the freedom, confidence, and support to make it happen.

Additional special thanks to my business partner and co-owner of RopeSport, David Schockett, who has made major financial and creative contributions over the years; Kelly Packard and Eric Nies, two well-known celebrities who starred in our series of workout tapes and are important parts of our team; Maya Joko and Jeremy Broffman, the two principal models in this book; Tony Ferro, principal photographer and jump-roper extraordinaire;

Eleanor Schockett, who has contributed greatly and been patient to a fault; Howard Frumes, an attorney who has given us excellent legal representation and advice for many years; Sheila Higgins, a wonderful director and coproducer of our workout tapes; David Lewine, who guided us through a number of difficult negotiations with honor, skill, and intelligence; Paul Goldberg, who saw RopeSport's marketing potential before almost anyone else; Kimberly Kim, a talented designer who provided invaluable help with certain illustrations; Kristin Borg of Borg Design Group, a fantastic graphic designer; and Joel Brokaw of the Brokaw Group, a public relations expert and true friend of RopeSport. All of these individuals have played an important role in making RopeSport what it is today, and I'm proud that many of them became friends as a result of our work together. A lot of them continue to help in innumerable ways that go far beyond what I could ever have hoped for, and for that I'll be eternally grateful.

Special gratitude to world leading fitness expert Kathy Smith for her support. In an industry plagued with far too many expensive gimmicks and so-called experts, Kathy stands out as a shining example of someone with true integrity as reflected in everything she does. Her tapes and books have helped improve the health and wellness of literally millions of people.

I also want to shout out a huge thanks to the many jumpers who have taken the RopeSport classes we teach over the years. A lot of the instructional techniques and information contained in this book came directly from jumping with you on a regular basis. It is no exaggeration to say that this book would not have been possible without your participation, enthusiasm, and support.

Finally, I want to say thank you to my family and friends. I know it's an oft-used cliché, but words truly can't express how I feel about you.

With so many people to thank, I've undoubtedly forgotten someone, so to all of you, a special thank-you.

RopeSport™

RopeSport™

The Ultimate Jump Rope Workout

Martin Winkler

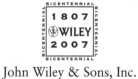

John Wiley & Sons, Inc.

Published by John Wiley & Sons, Inc., Hoboken, New Jersey
Published simultaneously in Canada

Photo credits appear on page 223 and constitute an extension of this copyright page.

Wiley Bicentennial Logo: Richard J. Pacifico

Design and composition by Navta Associates, Inc.

The information contained in this book is not intended to serve as a replacement for professional medical advice. Any use of the information in this book is at the reader's discretion. The author and the publisher specifically disclaim any and all liability arising directly or indirectly from the use or application of any information contained in this book. A health care professional should be consulted regarding your specific situation.

For general information about our other products and services, please contact our Customer Care Department within the United States at (800) 762-2974, outside the United States at (317) 572-3993 or fax (317) 572-4002.

Wiley also publishes its books in a variety of electronic formats. Some content that appears in print may not be available in electronic books. For more information about Wiley products, visit our web site at www.wiley.com.

Library of Congress Cataloging-in-Publication Data:

Winkler, Martin, date.
   Ropesport : the ultimate jump rope workout / Martin Winkler.
      p.   cm.
   Includes bibliographical references and index.
   ISBN 978-0-470-03631-0 (pbk.)
 1. Rope skipping.   I. Title.
   RA781.15.W562   2007
   613.7'10284—dc22   2006036224

Printed in the United States of America

10 9 8 7 6 5 4 3 2 1

Contents

Acknowledgments   vii

Introduction   1

PART I

Jump Start: An Introduction to RopeSport

1	The Top-10 Benefits of Jumping Rope	11
2	General Information and Background	16
3	Frequently Asked Questions	21
4	Getting Started	25
5	Learning How to Jump	33
6	RopeSport Philosophy and Style of Jumping	41
7	RopeSport Workout Format	45
8	RopeSport Fundamentals	55
9	Rope Turns	62

PART II

Jump In: Exercises That Take You through Beginning, Intermediate, Advanced, and Extreme Moves and Workouts

10	Basic Jumps	73
11	Basic Jump Combinations	83
12	Basic RopeSport Workouts	96
13	Intermediate Jumps	107
14	Intermediate Jump Combinations	116
15	Intermediate RopeSport Workouts	134
16	Advanced Jumps	146

17   Advanced Jump Combinations   153

18   Advanced RopeSport Workouts   172

19   Extreme Jumps   189

PART III

Jump Out: The RopeSport Way to a Healthier Lifestyle

20   Alternative RopeSport Workouts   197

21   Stretching   205

22   Strength Training, Muscle Toning, and
     Shaping   212

23   RopeSport for Fitness Professionals 217

24   Effective Training and a Healthy Lifestyle   220

Photo Credits   223

Index   225

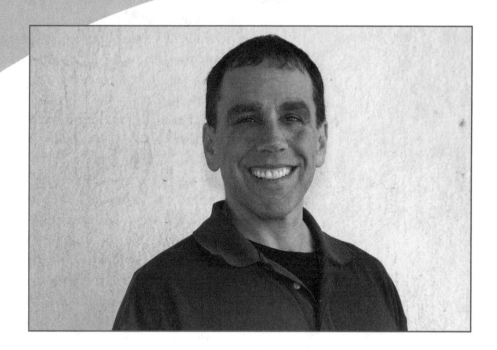

Introduction

Like so many millions of people, my first memories of jumping rope are as a kid on the local school playground. I remember it being a fun but short-lived experience, something I stopped doing by about the sixth grade. A lot of years would pass before I picked up a jump rope again.

In high school I played a number of sports, including basketball, ice hockey, and tennis. At that time the only training I did was specific conditioning exercises for the individual sport I was playing. Working out for general fitness and a healthy lifestyle wasn't part of the equation. During my college years I began to visit the gym fairly often. A typical workout would consist of playing a little pickup basketball, running a few times around an indoor track, and lifting a few weights. I still wasn't particularly serious or knowledgeable about fitness or nutrition.

After graduating from the University of California at Berkeley, I moved to Los Angeles, where *everyone* seemed to be working out. Due to the Hollywood entertainment industry's emphasis on looking good, the gym business was flourishing. It was at that time that I got serious about my own training; twenty years later I still spend a lot of my waking hours in the gym. Since I've been living in Los Angeles, a number of workouts have gained popularity, including aerobics, step, cardio boxing, spinning, yoga, and boot camp. At one time or another I've tried every one of these workouts and found all of them to be beneficial to some degree. In fact, it's my strongly held belief that *whatever* workout that's safe and motivates you to exercise on a regular basis is a very good thing. It was during this period that I rediscovered jumping rope.

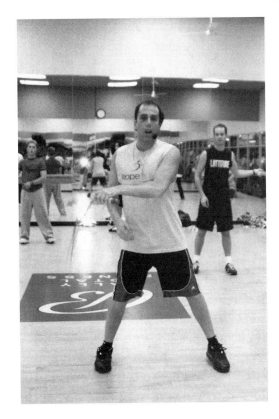

I am now in my forties and feel almost as healthy and strong as I did twenty years ago. During this twenty-year period I've also been able to maintain a consistent weight of 160 to 170 pounds. Equally as important, although I work out very intensely I have experienced no significant injuries. In fact, in some ways I am actually in *better* shape than I was twenty years ago. How have I been able to accomplish this? There is one simple answer: by doing the RopeSport jump rope workout on a regular basis.

Although I believe there are numerous workouts that are physically beneficial, I am convinced that the RopeSport jump rope program is far and away *the most* beneficial workout in existence. It is also the most fun. Minute for minute, there is simply no comparison.

By the time you finish this book I think you'll agree that the RopeSport jump rope program is absolutely phenomenal. Most importantly, you'll have learned the tools to begin your own RopeSport workout program. I guarantee you won't regret it.

About RopeSport

RopeSport LLC is a company dedicated to the sport of jumping rope: exercise that's fun, fat-blasting, and accessible to *everyone*. The name RopeSport also describes the style of jumping rope—a freestyle form that combines traditional jumping rope with music, dance, and natural body movements. People around the world love to jump rope. It's not only entertaining, but it's also one of the most effective ways to lose weight and get fit. That's why many elite fitness professionals, athletes, coaches, and trainers will tell you that RopeSport is one of the best cardiovascular cross-training workouts in existence.

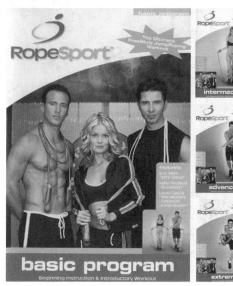

Through the use of an easy-to-follow, step-by-step teaching method I developed after years of working with thousands of beginning jumpers, almost anyone can learn to jump rope in only a few workouts.

RopeSport has been featured in numerous magazines and newspapers, as well as on a number of nationally known television shows. Our résumé includes appearances on *The Today Show* and *The View*, and features in *Cosmopolitan*, the *New York Times*, *Shape*, *Men's Health*, *GQ*, *Mademoiselle*, *Men's Fitness*, the *Los Angeles Times*, *Self*, and the *Washington Post*, to name a few.

RopeSport's goal is to teach millions of people throughout the world how to jump rope. We currently market a line of premium-quality jump ropes, award-winning workout DVDs, music CDs, and jumping mats. While the descriptions of the jumping techniques contained in this book are clear, watching our DVDs will make the

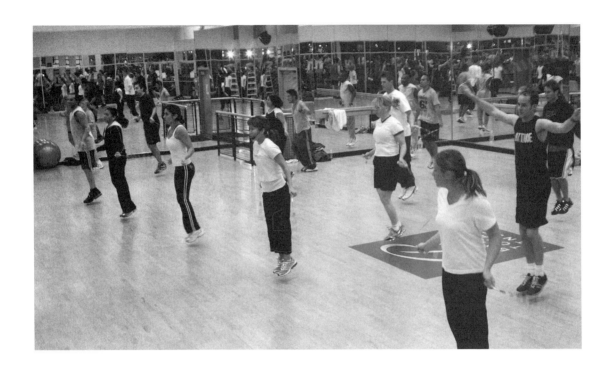

instructions that much easier to follow—I'd highly recommend it. For more information on RopeSport products or educational services, please visit www.ropesport.com.

Welcome to Jumping Rope

When you think of jumping rope there are very possibly two images that come to mind. First, you might think of boxers: well-conditioned athletes who use jumping rope as an indispensable part of their training routines. Second, maybe you think of kids jumping rope on the local school playground, something that millions of us (including me) did when we were younger.

What might *not* come to mind is that virtually anyone—including you—can become a proficient jump-roper in only a few workouts. Let me say it again in case there's any doubt: *you can and will learn to jump rope in just a few short workouts.*

The main obstacle to learning how to jump rope is that there has never been a detailed, easy-to-follow teaching method available to the general public—at least until now. Instead, most people are given a rope (a lousy one at that) and told to "go ahead and jump," with no further instruction. As a result, beginners often use an enormous amount of excess, unnecessary energy and become extremely winded in the matter of a few minutes. Additionally, they continue to get tangled in the rope, commonly referred to as "missing." Unfortunately, this frustrating experience causes far too many people, even those in good physical condition, to simply give up.

Well, no more.

After years of teaching thousands of people to jump rope, I've developed a unique, step-by-step teaching method that allows people of all shapes and sizes to become proficient jumpers in only a few workouts. In a nutshell, RopeSport utilizes the time-tested training principles of *active rest*, *interval training*, and *modifications* (these terms are explained later) so that almost anyone— regardless of their current level of physical condition—can learn to jump rope.

Success Story

Norman Eichel, 70, Real estate consultant

The RopeSport program is an amazingly easy way to stay in shape. I can't think of a better exercise program that's more fun than jumping rope. Last year I climbed Mount Kilimanjaro, and it helped get me ready for the climb.

About six years ago I got a new aortic valve, and my doctor wanted me to start exercising. He suggested jumping rope as one good way to get in shape and to take care of my ticker. It's fun. It's like dancing, that's why it's fun. There's music, you're free-flowing, and you're expressing yourself physically and emotionally. It's freedom of expression.

I think one of the fortunate events of my life was meeting Marty Winkler, who got me started in this whole thing. So as a mentor and a teacher, I owe him a great deal.

A good analogy is swimming. Virtually anyone can learn how to swim if they receive some good basic instruction. However, if you're just thrown into a pool with no instruction whatsoever, call the paramedics. The same is true for jumping rope.

If you're trying to find an effective, fun way to burn tons of calories and tone your entire body, you need look no further than RopeSport.

Who Can Jump?

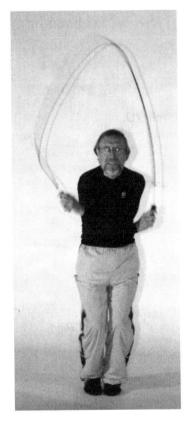

Everyone!

Over the years I've taught thousands of people to jump rope. Many of these same people came into class the first time wondering if they'd be able to successfully complete a one-hour jump rope class. They quickly found that the answer was a resounding yes. Whether you're age seven or seventy, in great shape or not, after finishing this book you will have all the information you need to become a proficient jumper in only a few workouts.

Men and Women

Maybe men identify with the image of a boxer who really knows how to work a rope. Maybe women have fond memories of jumping with their friends at school. Maybe it's because jumping rope burns an incredible amount of calories and fat in a short period of time. Whatever the reason, both sexes love to jump rope equally, something that's highly unusual when compared to many other workouts that appeal primarily to men *or* women, but definitely not both.

Kids

Kids absolutely love to jump rope! With childhood obesity and diabetes at virtually epidemic levels, RopeSport can make a major difference in the health and wellness of millions of kids throughout the world. Over the years I have done numerous demonstrations for K–12 schools, Parks and Recreation programs, and others, and the enthusiasm that RopeSport generates in these environments is a sight to behold. As far too many parents know, it can be an extraordinarily difficult task to get their kids up from in front of the television or computer. Jumping rope is simple and safe, an exercise that kids of all athletic abilities can participate in. It can be practiced individually or in a group, and it's so incredibly fun that kids find it self-motivational. The RopeSport style of jumping is heavily influenced by music and dance, and I've often described it as "MTV with a jump rope." The speed, sound, and power of the rope also make it visually dynamic, something that kids find really cool.

Recreational and Competitive Athletes

Many world-class athletes use RopeSport as an integral part of their training and believe it's an important reason for their success. From recreational soccer to competitive athletics, the skills that jumping rope develops will enhance athletic performance in almost any sport. In terms of staying in top physical condition all year round, it's hard to imagine a more beneficial exercise than jumping rope on a regular basis. That's why professional boxers swear by it.

Seniors and Sedentary Individuals

As it's traditionally been taught, jumping rope can be a strenuous activity. However, because RopeSport's unique teaching method utilizes a variety of easier modifications and equipment options, virtually anyone can participate—including senior citizens and sedentary individuals—and still enjoy its many benefits.

How to Use This Book

The way to use this book most effectively is to first read the whole book from beginning to end *before you start jumping*. Then go back and read it again. This time, however, when you get to a section of the book that gives you specific jumping instructions, pick up your jump rope and practice what's discussed in that section before you go on to the next section. Don't spend too much time on any particular jump or move if you're finding it difficult—just continue to a different jump without getting frustrated. Later on in your workout, or during your next workout, you can go back to whatever jump you found challenging.

As a general rule, I recommend practicing any individual jump for a *maximum* of 5 to 10 minutes before moving on to something else. If you approach your workouts this way, you'll learn most jumps within a few practice sessions. After you've learned just a few of the many jumps and techniques taught in this book you'll be ready to put together an effective, beneficial workout (see chapter 8, "RopeSport Fundamentals"). From that point on, while you continue to work out regularly you'll gradually add more jumps and progress to lengthier, more difficult workouts.

Part I

JUMP START

An Introduction
to RopeSport

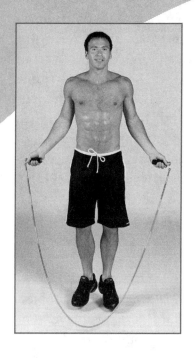

Chapter 1

The Top-10 Benefits of Jumping Rope

Many leading experts, including coaches, trainers, strength and conditioning experts, competitive athletes, and fitness professionals, believe that minute for minute, jumping rope is one of the most beneficial exercises a person can participate in. It is an unparalleled cardiovascular workout that will tone and strengthen your entire body.

Here are the top-10 reasons to jump.

1. Jumping Rope Burns up to a Thousand Calories an Hour

Because you're utilizing all the major muscle groups of your entire body, both upper and lower, you will burn an incredible amount of fat during your RopeSport workout—up to a thousand calories an hour! That's more calories than virtually any other exercise in existence and something that makes RopeSport truly unique. Even a 15-to-20-minute workout will burn lots of fat and help improve your overall fitness level.

2. Jumping Rope Will Tone Your Entire Body

Jumping rope is a fantastic exercise for shaping all the major muscle groups of the lower and upper body. Beginning with the lower body, jumping rope will do wonders for your calves, quadriceps, hamstrings, and glutes (your butt). What you may not realize, however, is how the constant turning motion of the rope will also shape and tone the entire upper body, including your chest, back, deltoids (shoulders), forearms, biceps, and triceps. In fact, when just beginning your RopeSport jump rope program, you might be surprised at just how great an upper-body workout you're going to get. If you're trying to develop long, lean cut muscles from head to toe—the kind of body most people are looking for—the RopeSport workout is just what the doctor ordered.

3. Jumping Rope Is Easy to Learn

Throughout the years that I've taught thousands of people to jump rope, probably the single most frequent objection I've heard is "It's just too hard" or "You have to be in great shape" to jump rope. Well, nothing could be further from the truth. In fact, through the use of an innovative teaching technique based on what I call Resting Moves and the Three-Step Breakdown (see pages 36–37, 38–39), *virtually anyone can become a proficient jumper in only a few workouts*. I've taught students from seven to seventy years old, from weekend warriors to professional athletes. The constant emphasis to go at your own pace with specific and easy-to-follow techniques for modifying your workout allows beginning jumpers, as well as people who might not be in the best of shape, to have a successful and beneficial experience almost immediately. And because you'll get it right from the start, you'll have a lot of motivation to stick with the RopeSport program. Time and again I've seen people who had some doubt about their own ability become great jumpers in a matter of a few weeks. As an instructor, nothing could be more rewarding, and it's one of the main reasons I still love teaching after all these years.

4. Jumping Rope Will Make You a Better Athlete

Professional boxers, arguably the most well-conditioned athletes in the world, have used jumping rope as an indispensable part of their training routines for many years. Elite athletes from a variety of sports, including tennis, basketball, golf, volleyball, skiing, and football, credit at least part of their success to jumping on a regular basis. The primary reason for this is that jumping rope will lead to improvements in agility, hand-eye-foot coordination, explosiveness, vertical-jumping ability, hand and foot speed, fluidity of movement, and timing. These skills are essential to maximizing performance in almost any sport you can think of. You'll "float like a butterfly and sting like a bee."

5. Jumping Rope Is Extremely Portable and Inexpensive

All you need to begin your RopeSport workout is a jump rope and a 4-by-6-foot area to jump in. A room in the house, a gym, a backyard, and a park are all ideal for your RopeSport workout. And jumping rope is perfect for traveling—just throw a rope in your suitcase and you've got the greatest portable workout in existence.

You can start your RopeSport workout with just one inexpensive item—a jump rope. In comparison to other popular fitness items flooding the market—many of which are, in my opinion, nothing more than expensive

Success Story

Roy Werner, 48, Actor

What I've found is that the calorie-burning aspect of the Rope-Sport program is fantastic. It's helped me lean up and keeps me sharp. Working in television and film, you have a lot of downtime on the set. With RopeSport I just throw my rope into my suitcase and work out in my hotel room or right on the set. When I'm jumping in class you see everybody having a good time; everybody is a team and we all push each other and have a blast.

gimmicks—jumping rope is extremely affordable, no matter what your budget. That's also one of the main reasons why jumping rope is part of physical education curriculums in K–12 schools throughout the world; for very little cost, an entire school can begin a jump rope program.

6. Jumping Rope Looks Really Cool

If you've ever seen someone at the gym who really knows how to work a rope, no doubt you've noticed how it attracts a lot of attention. There's something about the speed, power, and sound of the rope that makes it visually dynamic and even mesmerizing to watch. The visual appeal of extreme performance jumping is one of the main reasons we've made a lot of television appearances. You'll be sweating bullets, but you'll never look better doing it.

7. Jumping Rope Can Be Done Individually or in a Group

Another great thing about jumping rope is that you can do it by yourself or with a group. That gives you more flexibility to decide what kind of workout you want. If you prefer training by yourself, go ahead and jump on your own. If you're the type who likes working out with other people, jump with your spouse or kids. Jump rope classes are also springing up at gyms all around the country. Classes are a great place to find other people who can motivate you and vice versa. In my experience, teaching one another tricks and the camaraderie you get from jumping with fellow ropers are beautiful things. And you just can't beat the enthusiasm that you'll find in a high-energy jump rope class.

8. Jumping Rope Appeals Equally to Men and Women

Men, who have traditionally been reluctant to participate in group exercise classes, are flocking to RopeSport. Maybe men like to imagine themselves as boxers in training? Or maybe they're attracted to the powerful and explosive nature of jumping? Whatever the reasons, the fact is that jumping rope is one of the only exercises that appeals equally to both sexes. In a RopeSport class it's not uncommon for a 50/50 ratio of men to women, something that's virtually unheard of in group exercise environments.

9. Jumping Rope Is Great for Kids

One of the truly wonderful and unique things about RopeSport is that *kids love it, too*! I often describe our style of jumping, FreeStyle JumpRoping, as "MTV with a jump rope." It's one of the only exercises that kids will automatically gravitate toward because they find it self-motivational. Throw a bag of ropes into a room full of kids and within minutes they'll be jumping and having a great time. With numerous studies concluding that children are far too sedentary, a major contributing factor to the virtual epidemic of childhood obesity and diabetes currently plaguing the United States (and much of the industrialized world), RopeSport can truly make a difference. It is a wonderful activity for the entire family—Mom, Dad, and the kids.

10. Jumping Rope Is Fun

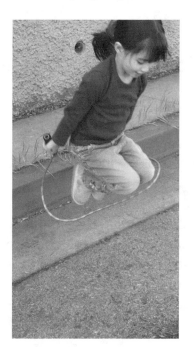

Last but definitely not least, jumping rope is incredibly fun! Due to the wide variety of jumps and tricks that you can incorporate into your workout, even as a beginner, your RopeSport workout will always stay challenging and motivational. Jumping rope appeals to the kid in all of us. Who doesn't have fond memories of jumping on the local school playground? It is a totally unique exercise in that it blends athleticism and art. It allows jumpers to be as creative as they want to be, whether it's inventing new jumps or jump combinations. And because you can always progress to a more advanced level, your RopeSport workout will never grow boring or monotonous. It really is a blast!

Chapter 2

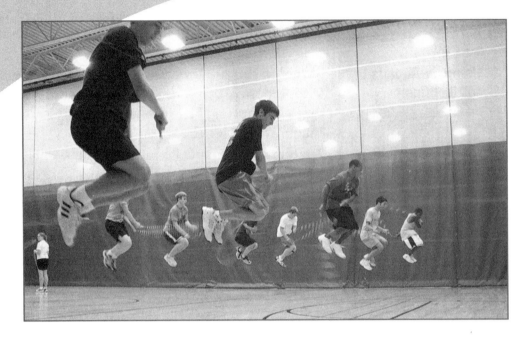

General Information
and Background

There are a lot of theories regarding the history and origins of jumping rope. One such theory holds that the Egyptians used to play a game where they'd cut a vine and jump over it. Others believe that jumping rope can be traced to festivals in ancient China. While I was traveling in the Netherlands a little over a year ago and shopping in a store that specialized in antique etched tiles (the Netherlands is famous for its tile work), I came across a tile dating back to the late 1600s that had a picture of a little boy jumping rope! We know that since the early 1900s boxers have used jumping rope as an important part of their training routines. About the same time, little kids began jumping rope on local school playgrounds. There are scenes of famous actors including Charlie Chaplin and Shirley Temple jumping rope in movies that were made well over fifty years ago. So one thing we can say with certainty is that jumping rope has been part of our popular culture for many years.

Styles of Jumping Rope

Double Dutch

Double Dutch is a style of jumping rope where there are two participants turning two ropes while either one or two participants jump through the ropes. Often associated with the inner city, Double Dutch is a dynamic form of jumping rope that kids really love. In addition to it being a beneficial cardiovascular exercise, Double Dutch also improves coordination and agility. Furthermore, because it requires three to four participants working closely together, it's also great for developing teamwork and cooperative skills among children. At the most advanced levels, Double Dutch is also being done as an extreme competition sport where groups of kids are doing high-energy choreographed routines that are sure to amaze. The two largest organizations that specialize in Double Dutch are the National Double Dutch League and the American Double Dutch League.

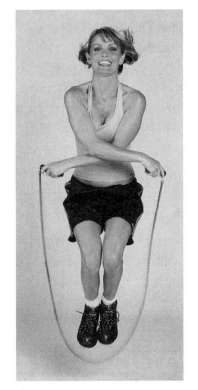

Single-Rope Jumping

Single-rope jumping is done by one person using one jump rope. It is the style of jumping rope that is the focus of this book. RopeSport is single-rope jumping.

In addition to the numerous physical benefits that you'll get from jumping rope on a regular basis, one of the big advantages of single-rope jumping is that it takes only one person to do it—you! And it doesn't require fancy or expensive equipment, just a piece of rope and two handles.

In fact, it's hard to imagine a piece of fitness equipment that's more basic than a simple jump rope. Interestingly, it is one of the least expensive forms of exercise you could choose to participate in, and it is also one of the most beneficial.

Ways to Jump

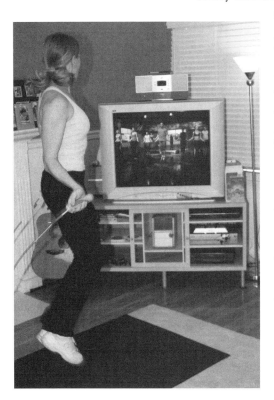

At Home   If you're someone who prefers to work out in the convenience of your own home, or you've only got thirty minutes to get in a workout, or you're a single parent without a babysitter, you can always jump rope at home. Your living room, basement, or backyard are all ideal for your workout. One advantage to jumping at home is that in addition to easily referencing information contained in this book, you have the option of jumping along with RopeSport's instructional DVDs or audio workout CDs.

Gyms   The gym is another great place to jump. If your gym has an aerobic floor with additional cushioning and support, so much the better. Combining jumping rope with weight training makes for an extremely effective workout that gives you the best of both worlds—cardio and strength training.

Office   If like many people these days the only time you have to work out is during your lunch break at work, your office is another place where you can jump.

Parks   If you like to work out outdoors, consider jumping at a local park. Another benefit of jumping at a park is there are other things for the kids to do—that is, if they're not already jumping rope with you!

Group Exercise Classes

If you're the kind of person who likes working out with other people, RopeSport group exercise classes are currently being taught at a number of gyms across the United States, including Bally Total Fitness. In a high-energy class where the ropes are flying, it's an absolute blast! There's also an element of friendly competition when students are showing off the latest tricks they've learned and motivating one another to work harder. As a beginning jumper, having the guidance of a qualified instructor is another big plus to jumping in class.

Jump Rope Teams

While primarily for kids, jump rope teams are springing up in many areas across the country. The leading organization for these teams is the United States Amateur Jump Rope Federation (www.usajrf.org). These teams are a great way to get your kids active by jumping in a supervised and supportive group setting. Jump rope camps and team competitions are held at certain times throughout the year. Extreme jumpers are pushing the sport to new limits with awe-inspiring tricks that seem to defy the laws of gravity. Most importantly, they are also learning about the benefits of a healthy, active lifestyle.

Jumping Rope Physiology 101

Let's briefly discuss how jumping rope affects your body and why.

Jumping rope requires the use of the muscles in both your upper and lower body. The turning motion of the rope involves all the major muscle groups of your upper body, including deltoids (shoulders), pectorals (chest),

Success Story

Jim Drewery, 52, Small-business owner

RopeSport burns a ton of calories and makes me feel light on my feet. It's low-impact and great for shaping my body. The teaching technique with the Resting Moves makes it easy to learn. It's also really fun. I love it.

biceps and triceps (arms), latissimus dorsi (back), and abdominals (stomach). The jumping motion requires the involvement of all the major muscle groups of your lower body, including quadriceps (front of thighs), hamstrings (back of thighs), gastrocnemuis and soleus (calves), and glutes (rear end). And because you're using the large muscle groups of your entire body to jump rope, your heart and lungs are being challenged and worked in a very big way. This makes jumping rope a phenomenal cardiovascular exercise that burns tons of calories and fat.

For the same reason that you're getting an excellent cardio workout—that is, you're using all your major muscle groups—you're also shaping and toning your entire body. This contrasts with a lot of other cardio exercises, including spinning and running, that focus mostly on your lower body.

If you're averaging 120 jumps or rotations per minute, a comfortable pace even for beginners, *in a 20-minute workout you've turned the rope and jumped off the ground well over two thousand times*. What's important about this is that the amount of resistance required for each individual jump is quite minimal. In contrast to low-repetition, high-resistance workouts like weight lifting that build bigger, bulkier muscles, jumping rope is fundamentally a low-resistance, high-repetition workout. It is the kind of exercise that develops lean, cut muscles from head to toe.

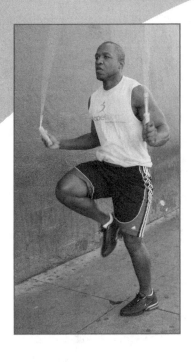

Chapter 3

Frequently Asked Questions

How does jumping rope compare to other forms of exercise?

Plainly and simply, jumping rope is very possibly the single most beneficial exercise you could participate in for improving your overall fitness level. It combines so many benefits, including maximizing cardiovascular conditioning, burning fat (up to a thousand calories an hour!), developing long, lean muscles, and optimizing athletic skills, that minute for minute, you just can't beat it. And all you need to get started is something as simple as a premium-quality jump rope.

Is it only for people in good shape or who are very coordinated?

Absolutely not. By using RopeSport's revolutionary teaching technique, jumping rope becomes so easy to learn that virtually anyone can become a proficient jumper in just a few workouts. We encourage people of all ages and fitness levels to give jumping rope a try—I guarantee you won't be sorry. In fact, I have a number of people over seventy years old who complete the one-hour classes I teach without stopping to take a rest—and they are absolutely phenomenal jumpers (not just for their age)!

Is it something my kids can do?

Yes! When introduced to them the RopeSport way, kids absolutely love to jump rope. In fact, jumping rope is one of the only exercises that kids take to naturally. Over the years I've done many presentations for K–12 schools and Parks and Recreation departments, and time and again it has warmed my heart to see how excited kids get when I put out a bag of ropes, turn on the music, and encourage them to jump in. With the tremendous increase in the levels of childhood obesity and diabetes in recent years, the fact that kids find jumping rope self-motivational is something of special importance to concerned parents.

How old does my child need to be to start jumping?

While it varies depending on your child's individual physical development, many kids can safely start jumping between the ages of six and eight. In general, kids need to have a basic level of coordination and strength to control the movement of the rope.

Is jumping rope too high-impact for many people?

Not if you're jumping with proper technique, where your feet are only leaving the ground a few inches. In fact, jumping rope can be practiced with far less impact than jogging. And for those people who have certain physical limitations, RopeSport utilizes modifications that make it very gentle on your body and keep you in complete control. However, while jumping rope is a very safe exercise, the minimal impact will help build strong bones and minimize any chance of osteoporosis, something that's especially important for a lot of women as they mature.

Isn't jumping rope boring and monotonous?

RopeSport teaches you such a large variety of jumps and tricks—even at the beginning level—that you'll always be able to challenge yourself, stay motivated, and have a

**Paul Rosenberg, 73,
Real estate agent**

As you get older, it's really beneficial to jump on a regular basis. You maintain your balance and your agility, and it keeps me feeling young. I run a lot also, and RopeSport is a perfect complement to my running. I just really enjoy it.

blast. And if you're like many people who like to work out to music, I highly recommend jumping to whatever kind of music motivates you, something that definitely keeps you pumped up and having fun.

I prefer to jump at home. Do I have enough room to jump indoors?

Yes. The jump rope only passes about two feet over your head, so there's enough room to jump in almost any living room. Your backyard, garage, or basement are all good places for your RopeSport workout. Another option is to do the workout by miming without the rope or by just using the handle—you'll get many of the same benefits.

I don't have a lot of time to dedicate to exercise. How long do I need to jump for?

You can get a great RopeSport workout in only 15 to 20 minutes. Combine it with some push-ups and sit-ups and you've got a complete, total body workout.

Can I add jumping rope to my current fitness routine?

Absolutely. RopeSport makes a great addition to virtually any exercise, including step aerobics, spinning, jogging, and lifting weights. It's an incredibly effective training tool to add to your workout arsenal.

How long should I jump for to get a good workout?

This is a question I'm asked a lot. In general, I'd recommend that you start with 20-minute workouts two to three times a week. Try it for a few weeks and if you feel comfortable, consider increasing the duration and frequency of your workouts. However, I really hesitate to give a one-size-fits-all answer because there are a number of factors that vary greatly from person to person including age, current level of physical condition, and how coordinated a person is. Further, because RopeSport teaches you how to modify your workout so you are in complete control over how much energy you are using, it is possible for beginners to work out for far longer than 20 minutes. In fact, over the years I've seen literally thousands of people complete a 1-hour RopeSport class their very first time! As with any new workout, remember to stretch (see chapter 21) and listen to your body. Safety is always your number-one priority.

Chapter 4

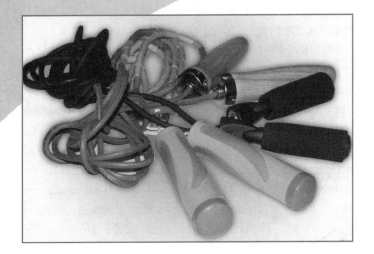

Getting Started

Before you embark on your RopeSport workout, let's make sure you've got the right equipment so that your workout is safe and fun, and you maximize the benefits in the shortest amount of time possible. After all, isn't that what most people are looking for from their workout? Quality equipment equals a quality workout, so let's be sure to jump in the right way.

Jump Ropes

The selection of a premium-quality jump rope can make a big difference in your RopeSport workout. You should consider the following.

Jump Rope Features

Adjustable Length   It's very important that your rope be adjustable in length so you can customize it to the exact length that's right for your height. In other words, someone who's six feet tall shouldn't be using the same-length rope as someone who's five feet tall. The reason it's important to have the right-size rope is that it will allow your arms to be in the correct jumping position. In turn, if your arms are in the correct position, it will allow you to rotate your rope with an energy-efficient motion, something that's essential to jumping with proper form and technique.

As your skill level increases and you become a more proficient jumper, you'll probably want to use a shorter-length rope than when you first started jumping, so having a rope that's adjustable will also let you shorten your rope without having to go out and buy a new one. The reason for graduating to a shorter rope is that it will give you greater control and maximize rotation speed for more-advanced jumps. The bottom line is that you'll get tired much faster than necessary by using a rope that's not the right length for your height, so make sure you're using a rope that's adjustable in length.

Minimized Twisting and Tangling   Another important feature of a good rope is that it's designed to minimize the tendency of the rope to twist or tangle. As a result, the rope will keep what we call a "true arc" and maximize the space you have to jump through it, thereby decreasing the chance of it catching on your feet or what is commonly referred to as "missing." You can determine if your rope will tangle a lot by holding the grips and letting it dangle— if it keeps a good shape you're ready to go. When the rope catches on a jumper's feet, quite often it has nothing to do with his or her technique. Rather, it's because the rope is constantly twisting and tangling. In a nutshell, if your rope is keeping a good shape, you'll have more space to jump through it and less chance you'll miss.

Handle Design   The last important feature you need to consider in selecting your rope is the handle design. First, you want a rope that has quality grips that feel comfortable in your hands, with good ergonomics. Second, a well-constructed handle results in a smooth, fast rotation and gives you complete control over the turning motion of the rope. Finally, you might also want to consider a rope

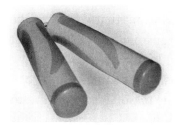

that has a removable cord so you can jump with the handles only, a modification that allows virtually anyone—sedentary, uncoordinated, and so on—to get a great workout right from the start.

Jump Rope Types

You can get a good workout with a variety of different materials and types of jump ropes. However, I definitely believe that some choices are better than others, and you should be well informed before you decide what kind of rope you're going to jump with.

Plastic-Beaded or Segmented Ropes   This is the type of jump rope I use during most of my workout, and it's what I often recommend for all-purpose jumping. The main reason I recommend plastic-beaded ropes is that the shape and weight of the beads cause them to twist and tangle less than ropes made from other materials. Plainly and simply, if your rope is keeping a good shape or true arc, there's less chance you'll miss. A beaded rope also gives you a great feel for the turning motion and rotation action of the rope.

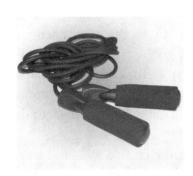

Speed Ropes   Speed ropes come in a variety of materials, but I've found steel-coated wire and PVC cord to be the fastest. In general, speed ropes are lighter than other ropes. The big advantage of using a well-designed speed rope is that it will give you maximum rotation speed, something that's very helpful when you're trying to execute more-advanced jumps. The downside, however, is that because they tend to be on the lighter side, they twist and tangle more often than a beaded rope. And a word of caution about speed ropes: because the rope is moving at a very fast speed, it might sting a little when you miss.

Leather Ropes   A lot of boxers train with leather ropes and swear by them. Similar to a speed rope, because they're a little on the light side they tend to twist and tangle a little more. If you're feeling like Rocky, give it a shot!

Weighted Ropes If you're trying to focus on upper-body development, weighted ropes will definitely give you a killer upper-body workout. However, I normally recommend using a weighted rope only if you've been jumping for a while and have reached a certain level of proficiency. Remember that jumping rope is extremely beneficial for all the major muscle groups of the upper body (biceps, triceps, chest, back, and deltoids), and jumping with a weighted rope increases the resistance and makes it an intense workout. Furthermore, because the increased weight causes the rope to rotate more slowly, the variety of jumps and tricks you can do will be limited.

Determining the Proper Length of Your Jump Rope

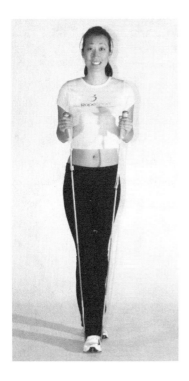

Start by gripping the handles as you would ski poles. Now put one foot—not two—on the center of the rope and pull up until the slack is out of the rope. The handles should come to just about the center of your chest; if they extend past your armpits the rope is definitely too long.

As you become a more-proficient jumper and you're progressing to more-advanced jumps and tricks, try shortening your rope a few inches and see if it helps. The reason for this is that *a shorter rope rotates faster*, something that's helpful in executing jumps like Doubles (where the rope rotates two times per jump).

Remember that having a rope that's the proper length will allow your arms to be in the correct position so you'll be turning the rope smoothly and efficiently. And that's what it's all about—developing an energy-efficient jump so you'll be able to train longer and get a fat-blasting, total-body workout.

In sum, time and again I've walked into a gym and seen people who were perfectly capable of learning to jump, but because they were using a poor-quality rope they were expending a huge amount of unnecessary energy and getting frustrated, one step away from giving up (or hanging themselves with the rope!). Using a premium-quality rope will serve to maximize your fun and minimize your learning curve. The bottom line is that it costs far less for a premium-quality rope than for a decent pair of sneakers, so why wouldn't you want to use the best rope possible?

Apparel

As far as shoes are concerned, I recommend that you use a good pair of cross-trainers or aerobic shoes. They should have good padding on the ball of the foot and be designed with lateral-movement support.

Workout clothing should be lightweight and form-fitting (not too baggy) so it doesn't catch on the rope. Materials that breathe are best for regulating your body temperature. As a beginning jumper you should consider wearing long workout pants and shirts that don't expose a lot of skin. That way when you hit yourself with your rope—something that happens a lot more often as a beginner—you'll have maximum skin protection. This is especially true for people with fair skin. In addition, women should consider wearing a supportive sports bra—for example, the type used by runners works well.

Hair

Women or men with long hair should wear a cap or put it up so it doesn't catch on the rope.

Music

If you like to work out to music, you can jump to any style that motivates you, including contemporary dance, rock, hip-hop, and country. They're all great to jump to. However, whatever type of music you decide on, it's very important that it's formatted at the right tempo.

The tempo of the music is important because it will help you to turn the rope at the right speed, guaranteeing that you'll get an awesome cardiovascular workout. Also, turning the rope either too slow or too fast can cause a variety of problems—because jumping rope really is about rhythm and timing, the music will actually help you to jump with proper technique.

For beginning jumpers, the correct tempo is 120 to 125 beats a minute. For intermediate jumpers, it's 125 to 130 beats a minute. For advanced jumpers, it's 130 to 135.

And when you've become an advanced jumper (that's right, I'm talking to you!) and are trying to really push yourself by "interval training," or sprinting with the rope, 160 beats a minute is definitely doable.

As a general rule, try to jump over the rope one time for each beat of the music. When you're first starting to jump, however, it's only natural for the music to feel a little fast. As a beginning jumper it's perfectly fine to jump slower and turn the rope at whatever speed you're comfortable with. Try not to push yourself too hard if you're feeling overly winded, but eventually you want to work toward jumping to the beat of the music.

Personally, I love to crank up the music when I'm in a space where the volume isn't an issue. Time just flies by when a great song is playing—it helps you to train longer and get that killer workout. In the classes I teach I'll periodically yell out, "You're just dancing with your rope," and there's no doubt that we all dance better when there's music playing that really motivates us. Just find a style of music that makes you want to get up and move.

You can purchase professionally designed music that's formatted at specific, consistent tempos without breaks between songs.

Jumping Mats

Some people like to use jumping mats to protect their carpets or floors. A good-quality mat will also give you extra cushioning and support for your knees and lower back. If you decide to buy a mat, make sure it's at least 3 feet by 4 feet, large enough to fully cover the swing of the rope. You also want a mat with some give but that's not too mushy, or you'll sink down too far and it'll be difficult to jump back up. In addition to jumping, you can also use a mat to do floor work such as push-ups, sit-ups, and stretching.

Safety

As with any exercise or workout, safety is paramount, and I always advise new jumpers to consult with a doctor before beginning any exercise program. This is especially true if you have some type of preexisting injury or medical condition.

Hydration

You've got to drink a lot of water before, during, and after your workout. Remind yourself to take water breaks at regular intervals during your workout. After training for as many years as I have I'd like to think I've learned a thing or two, and at the top of my priority list is drinking a *minimum* of eight to ten glasses of water each and every day. There is no doubt in my mind that it will help you to train longer, with more intensity, and with faster recovery.

Modifications

Always be sure to work at your own pace and difficulty level—who cares what the person next to you is doing? Remember that you can still burn a ton of fat and calories and get a great workout without doing the most advanced jumps and tricks. Conversely, if you're feeling strong on any given day or trying to take your RopeSport workout to the next level, consider pushing yourself harder by incorporating more of the advanced jumps and techniques, or just jumping longer.

Breathing

Breathing properly while you're jumping, and for that matter working out in general, is very important and something that most people don't give much thought to. However, it can make a big difference in how long and intensely you train. It is something that's important, and it shouldn't be taken for granted. The following suggestions stem in large part from the breathing techniques commonly used in meditation and yoga, other disciplines I practice on a regular basis that are excellent complements to your RopeSport workouts.

While you're jumping, try to stay connected with your breathing. Be in touch with each individual breath. Feel the air entering your body during the entire inhale. Feel how your stomach expands. On the exhale, be in touch with the feeling of the air leaving your body and how your stomach contracts. I'm not talking about *thinking* about your breathing, but rather about *feeling* it entering and leaving your body.

If you remind yourself regularly during your workout to connect with your breathing, your respiratory system will regulate itself more efficiently. In turn, your breathing will be more controlled and even. And although you're engaged in a relatively strenuous activity like jumping rope, you won't be using *unnecessary* energy beyond what is needed for your workout. In simple terms, you'll feel far less winded when you're breathing properly, enabling you to train longer and harder.

The talk test is a simple yet effective method to monitor your breathing. While you're jumping, you should be able to have a conversation with someone. I'm referring to stringing a few short sentences together, not a lengthy discourse about the meaning of life. If you're huffing and puffing so hard that you can't even yell "Help," then you're working too hard and need to move to a different jump or technique that requires less expenditure of energy (much more on this later). Conversely, if your breathing is so relaxed that you can talk nonstop for 15 minutes about how your last boyfriend or girlfriend was a total jerk, you should consider increasing your intensity level so you're breathing a little harder.

As simple as breathing properly may sound, it requires conscious work and practice. This is even truer during an activity like jumping rope, when your heart rate and adrenaline are pumping, your metabolism is greatly increased, and you're working hard. Most people's minds are constantly wandering from the past to the future, not connected in a meaningful way with what's happening here and now. In turn, that's what makes being completely in touch with each individual breath as it enters and leaves your body far from simple.

Chapter 5

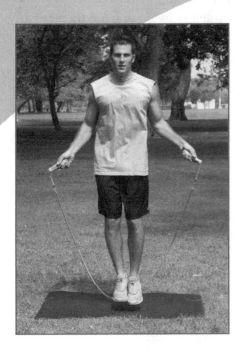

Learning How to Jump

Jumping with proper technique is extremely important. Without it, the effectiveness of your workout will be greatly diminished. Using proper form is the best way to minimize any chance of injury while allowing you to jump with the most energy-efficient motion possible, often referred to by fitness professionals as "economy of motion." Throughout your workout, remind yourself to focus on the fundamentals, no matter what jump you're doing or how tired you're feeling.

Proper Jumping Technique

The position of your arms and how you're turning the rope are critical components of proper jumping technique, so let's start there. You should be using some wrist and some forearm to turn the rope. Try to make small circles. (It might help to think of a cranking motion.) Be careful that you're using a combination of both wrist

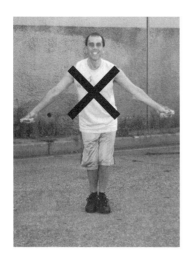

and forearm. In fact, one of the most common mistakes I've seen with beginning jumpers is that they'll turn the rope with their arms extended way away from their torso, using only their wrists with very little forearm. As a result, their shoulders do most of the work, and they get tired very quickly because of improper jumping technique.

Something else that causes the arms to extend away from your torso and into an incorrect jumping position is using a rope that's too long. It forces your arms to compensate for the improper length, while a rope that's sized properly allows the arms to remain in a natural, relaxed position. Again, you want to try to keep your elbows right by your torso and make sure that your forearms are angled toward the front, not extended out to your sides. If your arms are in the correct position and you're turning the rope with a balance of wrist and forearm, the result is a relaxed, energy-efficient rotation action. We refer to it as having a "smooth stroke," and it's something you should focus on from your very first workout.

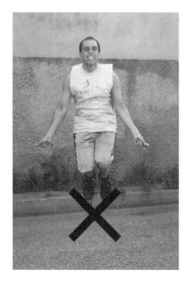

Another important part of proper jumping technique is only jumping a few inches off the ground, just enough room to let the rope pass under your feet. *Remember that jumping rope is about timing, not how high you jump.* Another common mistake I see with beginning jumpers is that they jump far too high off the ground. This causes them to use a lot of excess energy and to land with way too much impact. When you're jumping with proper form there is very little impact, much less than in many other aerobic activities and far less than running. As a beginning jumper, constantly remind yourself to land softly. Some mental imagery I've found helpful is to imagine you're jumping on a glass floor—if you land too hard, you break the floor.

Try to keep your shoulders down and relaxed, not up and tight. Your knees should remain soft and act like shock absorbers. You're pushing up off the balls of your feet and your heels are just tapping the ground. Your hands should stay level with your hips; don't let them rise up or the rope will catch on your feet. This is a common error when you're learning a new jump—while your body goes up, your hands should stay down.

One last thing we see with a lot of beginning jumpers is that they'll take an extra little jump or what we call the Bunny Hop. The basic rule of thumb when you're starting out is to take one jump per revolution of the jump, not two (there are some exceptions to this rule with certain advanced jumps—for example, *Doubles*, where the rope rotates twice per jump). There's nothing inherently wrong with the Bunny Hop. In fact, it's very gentle on the body, but it will limit your ability to execute a lot of different jumps and if possible should be avoided.

Usually the Bunny Hop is the result of turning the rope too slowly, causing you to take an extra jump while you wait for the rope to come around. A simple correction for the Bunny Hop is to just *turn the rope faster*. Try jumping to the beat of the music, and remember that having music formatted at the right tempo is very helpful.

PROPER FORM CHECKLIST

- Use some wrist and forearm when turning the rope. Make small circles or a cranking motion.
- Only jump an inch or two off the ground. Do not make big jumps.
- Try to land softly.
- Look straight ahead. Watching your feet doesn't help.
- Hands should stay level with the hips. Don't let them raise or lower.
- Push off and land with the balls of the feet. Heels should just tap the ground.
- Relax your neck.
- Shoulders stay down and relaxed. Avoid hunching.
- Keep your elbows bent and by your torso. A rope that's too long will pull your elbows away from your torso.

- Calves, quadriceps, and hamstrings act as shock absorbers.
- Turn the rope to the beat of the music (120 to 135+ beats per minute). Turning too slow or too fast causes problems.
- Remain loose but controlled.
- Breathe normally. You should be able to have a conversation with someone while you're jumping.

Do's	Don'ts
• Use some wrist and forearm to turn the rope.	• Don't turn the rope using only your wrists.
• Keep your elbows by your torso.	• Don't extend your arms out to the side.
• Only jump 2 to 3 inches off the ground.	• Don't jump too high.
• Make sure your rope is the proper length.	• Don't use a rope that's too short or long.
• Turn the rope to the beat of the music.	• Don't turn the rope too fast or too slowly.

Resting Moves and Recovery

Resting Moves are a central part of the RopeSport teaching technique and one of the principal ways that Rope-Sport differs from traditional jumping rope. You normally use Resting Moves after you've been jumping through the rope, are feeling winded, and need to bring your heart rate down. You want to catch your breath without coming to an abrupt stop and standing still. The way you accomplish this goal is surprisingly simple: *by slowly turning the rope to the side of your body*. In other words, by continuing to turn the rope to the side of your body with low-intensity Rope Turns you are recovering while still burning fat and calories. The most common Resting Moves are Figure 8s, 2 Turns to Each Side, and Step Touches.

By alternating between jumping through the rope and then recovering with the low-intensity Rope Turns and Resting Moves, you are using an effective training technique long advocated by fitness professionals and athletes

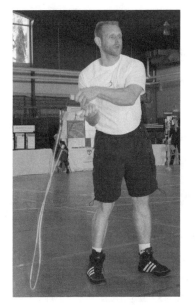

called "interval training." The lower-intensity periods where you're turning the rope to the side of your body with minimal expenditure of energy are also referred to as "active rest," meaning that you'll continue to receive cardiovascular benefits as long as you keep moving. Never feel that you need to keep up every step of the way; you can always modify your RopeSport workout and make it a little easier any time you're feeling overly winded and need a break. And that's how we get people who are taking class for the very first time—as well as a number of students of mine who are in their seventies—to complete a one-hour jump rope class!

Resting Moves and Rope Turns are also important for other reasons: they allow the beginning jumper to get comfortable with the turning motion of the rope without having to worry about jumping through it. Additionally, they are a safe, easy way to warm up your body with very little impact before you actually start jumping. Finally, they add variety to your workout.

Other Important Modifications

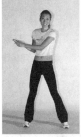

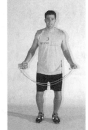

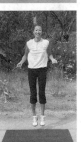

There are three additional modifications, all of which are variations on the same theme, that require less energy and coordination than jumping through the rope. At the same time, however, they are still highly beneficial. They are an integral part of the RopeSport teaching technique that every jumper should have in their jump rope arsenal.

1. Jumping with the Handles Only (with or without weights)
2. Jumping while Holding on to the Rope
3. Jumping without the Rope (miming)

These modifications are important for a number of reasons. First, they allow virtually anyone—sedentary, overweight, uncoordinated—to get many of the same benefits that you would by jumping through the rope. Let me repeat it: you get many of the same benefits jumping without the rope as you do with the rope. Further, no matter how strong and conditioned a roper you are, invariably there will be some period of time during your workouts when you're feeling really drained or winded, a perfect time to incorporate these modifications. In addition to requiring less expenditure of energy, there's no worry whatsoever about "missing," or catching the rope on your feet, so these moves are also great for the beginner who can be a little less coordinated. Furthermore, by jumping with any of these modifications you are in complete control over how much (or should I say how little) impact your body is getting, so they are very safe. And while almost any room has enough space and ceiling height to jump in, because the rope isn't rotating over your head these modifications can all be done in an extremely small area, a hotel room, for example. And finally, you're also practicing the timing and footwork that you need to execute the same jump, if and when you choose to jump through the rope. In sum, you can do the Basic 2 Foot Jump, the Alternating Foot, the Run, or the Straddle using any of these modifications—you'll still be getting the cardiovascular benefits, burning fat, learning the jump, and keeping it safe.

The Three-Step Breakdown

The Three-Step Breakdown is a teaching technique designed to help you master a wide variety of jumps by breaking the jump into its separate components. At the same time, you'll be executing the jump safely and with proper technique.

Start *step one* by putting the rope down and doing the Basic 2 Foot Jump without the rope. If you're using a rope with a removable cord, you can also do this by using only the handles. In other words, you're miming the jump without the rope. In turn, this will help you to learn the footwork and timing of the jump without having to worry about missing, or the rope catching on your feet.

Now let's focus on the position of your arms and the rotation action. Let your hands drop to your sides. Wherever they fall naturally is right about the position they

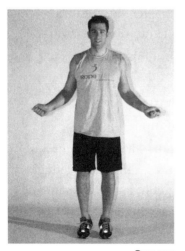

Step one

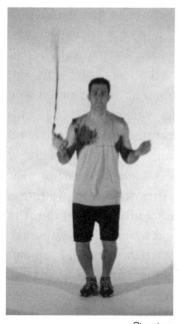

Step two

should be in when you're jumping. Your forearms are angled forward, not out to your sides. Now start jumping while you continue to mime the turning motion of the rope. Make sure your elbows stay by your torso and don't extend away from your body. The turning motion is a combination of wrist and forearm—make small circles or a cranking motion. You should only be jumping a few inches off the ground and landing softly with your whole body acting like a human shock absorber. Your shoulders stay down and relaxed, not up and tight. Try to breathe normally.

In *step two*, you add the rope by putting both grips in one hand and turning the rope to the side of your body at the 12 and 6 o'clock positions while you continue to do the Basic 2 Foot Jump. Try to make sure the rope doesn't drift to the right or to the left, but stays at 12 and 6 o'clock. This takes a little getting used to, and you might have to adjust the position of your wrist to keep the rope turning straight ahead. Try turning the rope at the same tempo and don't let it slow down or speed up. As with step one, you're still learning the foot-work and timing of the jump without having to worry about missing.

In *step three*, you execute the same Basic 2 Foot Jump through the rope.

In sum, the Three-Step Breakdown is a systematic way to learn any new jump. First you do it without the jump rope; then with the rope turning to the side of your body; then jumping through the rope.

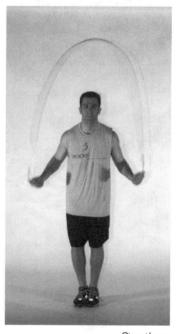

Step three

It's Okay to Miss

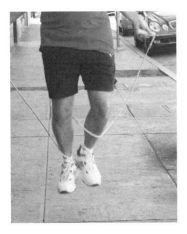

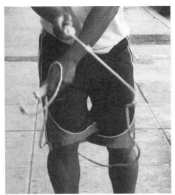

When the rope catches on your feet, in ropers' vernacular it's called "missing." Missing happens to everybody, beginners as well as experts, and it's a natural part of jumping, something to be expected during your workout. It's nothing to get frustrated or upset about (I've even seen people throw their rope after a few misses!), but rather it's no big deal and should be thought of as such. In fact, you might even try to look at missing in a positive light, a reminder that something is not quite right with your technique and that you need to practice a little more. Of course, missing happens more often when you're a beginner—the more skilled you become, the less you miss. Many moons ago, when I first started jumping, I remember watching more advanced jumpers and being amazed that they'd jump continuously for 30 to 60 minutes with only a few misses their entire workout!

Another time when you may experience frequent misses is when you're learning a new jump. If you're missing a lot, I suggest practicing the jump for a few minutes maximum and then moving on to a different jump. It's better to practice a new jump that's proving to be a little difficult for frequent, short periods of time, rather than continuing to practice the same jump until you reach the point at which you're frustrated. If you approach your workout this way, you'll master most jumps pretty quickly. Besides, there are so many different jumps with RopeSport, why get stuck on just one of them? The bottom line is that if you're not missing, you're not jumping rope.

Chapter 6

RopeSport Philosophy and Style of Jumping

Every person has his or her own natural and unique way of moving, and in some ways the most important thing I can teach you about the RopeSport jumping philosophy—and I can't stress this point enough—is that you get a sense of how to relax and move with the rope. Remember that it's not so much about how many tricks and jumps you can learn, but how you put them together in your own individual and creative style. The RopeSport style of jumping shares a lot of similarities with dancing— everyone moves and grooves with their own individual flavor. I sometimes tell students that the rope is their dance partner or remind them that they are dancing with their rope. Interestingly, these individual differences in style may be most apparent when students are executing a variety of Rope Turns to the side of their body in any order they want, referred to as FreeStyle Rope Turns. In other words, while a primary purpose of turning the rope to the side of

**Tom Henry,
52, Training
director**

I have a bad knee, and jumping rope is one of the only aerobic exercises I can do. I love the FreeStyle part of the class where you can just do your own thing and dance with the rope. If I jump a few times a week and keep a balanced diet, it's easy to stay lean.

your body is to recover and catch your breadth, it's also the time when students tend to get funky and even sexy, letting it all hang out. In the classes I teach, a lot of the time everyone is in unison doing the same jump at the same time, but part of the time we're just improvising on our own. And that's the FreeStyle element that everybody loves.

And because of the huge variety of jumps and moves you can incorporate into your workout—even as a beginning jumper—you'll always be able to challenge yourself and stay motivated by going from one jump to another, by going in and out of the rope with FreeStyle Jumps and Rope Turns, by transitioning from fast to slow and slow to fast, by creating thousands of different combinations. I've been working out for over twenty years and tried hundreds of different workouts, and to this day I can honestly say that I have never found any exercise that even comes close to RopeSport in terms of how physically beneficial it is. And in terms of pure fun, there's no comparison, either. Nothing feels quite as powerful as when you're loose and relaxed, the music's pumped up, you're just cruising from move to move, and you're sweating hard. There's nothing else like it. Athletes sometimes describe the euphoric feeling they have when performing at their absolute optimum level as being in the zone or the flow state, and I believe that jumpers experience this same feeling at times. The jump rope becomes an extension of your body and you're effortlessly executing tricks and moves without even trying. And that's why we call it RopeSport: The Ultimate Jump Rope Workout.

Going In and Out of the Rope

Alternating from jumping inside the rope to outside of the rope is a critical part of the RopeSport jumping style and philosophy. The truth is that if I had to jump through (or inside) the rope for my entire workout I'd get bored pretty fast. In fact, it's seldom that you'll see me jumping continuously through the rope for an extended period of time. Far more often I'm executing a

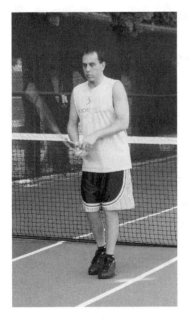

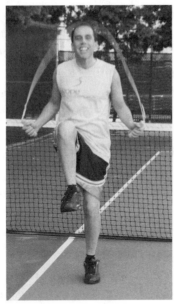

few different jumps through the rope; then I'm out of the rope; then I'm jumping through the rope again; then I'm out of the rope; then I'm in the rope; then I'm out of the rope. And I want to be clear I'm not talking about using the time that I'm out of the rope to recover and catch my breath. I'm talking about using FreeStyle Rope Turns because they add variety and are fun as heck. And that's how we do it the RopeSport way.

A great drill you should try is going in and then out of the rope as fast as you can. It'll make your Figure 8 Entrances and Figure 8 Exits as smooth as silk (see chapter 8, "RopeSport Fundamentals").

FreeStyle Soloing

This part of your workout in many ways defines what makes RopeSport different from traditional jumping rope. Plainly and simply, what you're doing when you FreeStyle is combining jumps and rope turns in any order you want for as long as feels good to you. Maybe you're going in and out of the rope. Maybe you're changing speeds from fast to slow and slow to fast. And maybe you're doing all of these things.

If you're a beginning jumper, your FreeStyling will consist of beginning Rope Turns and jumps. If you're a more advanced jumper, you'll probably incorporate a much wider variety of moves. Regardless of your skill level, however, it's important to remember that you can put together an awesome FreeStyle routine with only a few jumps and Rope Turns. It's about quality, not quantity.

I've seen beautiful FreeStyle routines consisting mostly of slow, graceful ballet-style Rope Turns. I've also seen awesome FreeStyling that consisted mainly of going in and out of the rope at lightning-fast speed with only a few different jumps, a style of jumping that I personally gravitate toward. I've seen extreme jumpers solo with jumps and tricks that will make your jaw drop. The point is that there's no one best way to FreeStyle. We all have our own individual style, and it's all good.

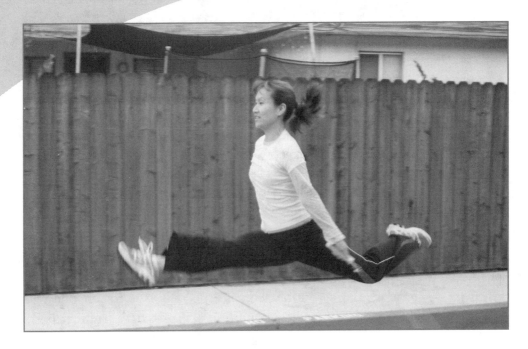

Chapter 7

RopeSport Workout Format

This chapter contains an overview of a complete Rope-Sport workout. The format is similar to most traditional group exercise classes that are taught in gyms, including warm-up, stretch, cardiovascular workout, strength training, cooldown, and flexibility segments. I strongly advise that you always do a warm-up and stretch before the cardiovascular portion of your workout, followed by a cooldown and stretch at the end. For safety reasons and to prevent injury, you need to stretch before and after every workout. It's also a good idea to consult

Pat Shannon, 42,
Sales representative

It's the most challenging cardio workout I've ever done. I'm not a natural athlete, and RopeSport has really helped improve my coordination. There's always something you can work on and take it to the next level. Every time I jump I'm thinking how I can improve and what I might do differently, and that's exciting. I also love the fact that the workout is so portable, you can take it anywhere. I do it in my house, I do it in my backyard, and I do it when I'm traveling. It's super convenient.

with a physician before embarking on any new exercise routine. This is especially true for anyone with a specific medical condition or a preexisting injury that could affect your workout. The strength training section is optional, although I definitely recommend it for the most effective total body workout with maximum fat-burning potential.

Preparation

Take time to prepare yourself for your workout. *It's very important to properly hydrate yourself by drinking a lot of water before, during, and after your workout.* Make sure to bring whatever music you plan on jumping to; I can't tell you how many times I've gotten to the gym and been really bummed out after realizing I'd forgotten my music. Have a towel so you can dry off when you begin to sweat. Bringing a dry shirt to change into at the end of your workout is also a good idea, especially if it's a cold day outside. You want to keep your muscles warm after you've trained hard.

Warm-up

The warm-up is a short period of activity at the very beginning of your workout where you combine Rope Turns and a few Basic Jumps in order to slowly elevate your heart rate and get your blood flowing throughout the entire body. You're preparing for the main cardiovascular portion of your workout with low- to moderate-intensity moves and jumps.

Start with some FreeStyle Rope Turns where you're turning the rope slowly to the side of your body with Figure 8s, 2 Turns to Each Side, and Step Touches, combining them in any order you want (see chapter 9). These FreeStyle Rope Turns are all very gentle on your body and an effective, safe way to begin your workout. After a few minutes, add the Figure 8 Bouncing. Continue with the Figure 8 Bouncing for a few minutes to really warm up your feet and legs. Make sure that your feet are barely leaving the ground while you're bouncing so the impact to your body is minimal. Remember this is just the warm-up, so resist the urge to start full speed or you'll tire far too quickly. You always want to start your workout slowly and *gradually* increase the speed and intensity of your workout. This will also minimize any chance of injury.

Once your upper and lower body feel loose and warm, begin to jump through the rope for short intervals of 30 to 45 seconds each. Use the 2 Foot Jump, the Alternating Foot, or a combination of both. Remind yourself to land softly.

After each short jumping interval, do another 30 to 60 seconds where you're going in and out of the rope. Use controlled, relaxed Figure 8 Entrances and Figure 8 Exits to go in and out of the rope. This is the beginning of some low-intensity FreeStyle Jumping.

Continue to alternate among Rope Turns, Basic Jumps, and FreeStyle for the remainder of the warm-up.

Stretch

Now that your body is warmed up, it's time to stretch. *It's very important to stretch adequately in order to minimize any chance of injury.* Stretching is a critical part of your workout that far too many people—especially men—don't spend nearly enough time on.

Throughout the stretch, be sure to connect with your breathing; a helpful technique commonly used in yoga is to imagine your breath going right into the specific muscle you're stretching. Don't force yourself deeper into the stretch, something that could result in a muscle pull. Rather, try to relax into the stretch, maybe going a little deeper with each exhale. Be sure to begin the stretch slowly and only go as far as you're comfortable, paying careful attention to how your body is feeling. Avoid bouncing when you're doing a particular stretch, commonly referred to as ballistic stretching. It can cause your muscles to tighten and lead to injury.

Water Break

After you've stretched all your major muscle groups from head to toe, take a short break to grab a drink of water. If you stop for more than a minute or two, your muscles will start to cool down and tighten up, defeating the purpose of the warm-up and stretch, so make it quick.

Get ready to sweat!

Jump Rope Cardio

Now that you've completed your warm-up and stretch, you've arrived at the main cardio portion of your workout. This is why you decided to give RopeSport a try, what it's all about.

In order for your workout to remain safe and effective, you should begin the cardio portion of your workout at a slow to moderate pace. You want to *gradually* increase your intensity level until you feel as if you're working really hard and expending a lot of effort at the peak of your workout. Toward the end of the cardio portion of your workout, it is very important that you spend a *minimum* of 2 to 3 minutes to bring your heart rate down safely by executing some low-intensity rope turns or Resting Moves. Coming to an abrupt stop and standing still immediately after you've jumped hard is something that causes a sharp drop in your heart rate and should be avoided for safety reasons. Be sure to take time to cool down properly.

FreeStyle Rope Turns

Get your blood flowing again and your heart rate up by beginning the cardio portion of your workout with a variety of FreeStyle Rope Turns done at a slow to moderate pace. Use any combination you'd like of low-intensity Figure 8s, 2 Turns to Each Side, or Step Touches. Get creative while continuing to turn the rope to the side of your body, either forward or backward. Stay with these FreeStyle Rope Turns for a few minutes.

Individual Jumps

The second part of your workout consists of executing a variety of individual jumps and Rope Turns. Choose from any of the beginner, intermediate, or advanced jumps and Rope Turns that you're comfortable with. As a general rule, beginners should do any individual jump for 16 to 32 counts or about 10 to 15 seconds. Intermediate or advanced jumpers should do any individual jump for 48 to 64 counts or 25 to 30 seconds. It's important to keep in mind, however, that these are very general guidelines. The actual length of time you jump will vary greatly depending on a number of variables, including the tempo at which you're jumping, how good shape you're in, and the difficulty level of the jump you've chosen. A good guide is to continue to do the jump until you've reached the point at which you need to catch your breath and recover by going back to the Resting Moves.

Resting Moves and Recovery

You use Resting Moves to catch your breath after you've been jumping through the rope for an extended period of time and need to temporarily decrease the intensity level of your workout. Remember that you can use these Resting Moves whenever you need to catch your breath. And if you should decide to stay with these low-intensity moves for a significant portion of your workout, that's perfectly fine! As long as you continue turning the rope, jumping with the handles, or holding on to the rope while you continue to bounce—that is, as long as you keep moving and don't stand still—you are burning fat and getting a lot of the same benefits you'd get from jumping through the rope. At the same time you're getting more comfortable with the turning motion of the rope, as well as learning the footwork and timing of a particular jump. So never hesitate to modify your workout and make it a little easier.

Sprint Interval Jumps

It's very beneficial to also include Sprint Intervals of 20 to 60 seconds each during your workout where you're jumping at close to your maximum speed. I normally start to incorporate Sprint Intervals 5 to 10 minutes into the workout. That way your heart rate is already elevated, but at the same time you've still got a lot of energy left to push really hard. The four most commonly suggested jumps for Sprint Intervals are the 2 Foot Jump, the Alternating Foot, the Run, and the Boxer Shuffle. However, as your skill level progresses, you can use almost any jump. The point of these Sprint Intervals is to push yourself really hard for short bursts in order to kick your metabolism into overdrive, thereby maximizing the cardiovascular benefits while burning tons of fat. This technique is commonly used by competitive athletes and I highly recommend it. Don't forget that even while you're jumping fast and the rope is flying, you should still be jumping with proper form and technique. Safety and injury prevention are always paramount.

Recovery Jumps

After you've completed a Sprint Interval, you're probably breathing hard. The next time you jump into the rope you should do what I refer to as a Recovery Jump. The primary purpose of a Recovery Jump is to keep your heart rate elevated, but at a less intense level, after you've worked at close to your maximum with a Sprint Interval. I use Recovery Jumps as a time to refocus on proper form and technique, and when jumping with an energy-efficient motion *you should be able to recover as you continue to jump through the rope*. With your heart rate racing after a Sprint Interval, you should also use this time to check in with your breathing.

Jump Combinations

In addition to doing individual jumps throughout your workout, you will also want to string together a variety of jumps into various combinations. It's basically the same thing that dancers do when performing a routine and is common in choreographed group exercise classes.

Creating jump combinations is just one more way to have fun, challenge yourself, and maximize the benefits of your RopeSport workout.

If you're a beginner, your combinations will consist of fewer jumps and you will repeat the sequence fewer times. For intermediate and advanced jumpers, you will incorporate a larger variety of jumps and/or repeat the sequence more times.

Long Jump

The Long Jump is used at the end of the cardio portion of your workout. It is analogous to jogging at a moderate pace for an extended period. The goal is to continue jumping through the rope the whole time if possible. Continue to work hard, but pace yourself at the same time. It's an ideal time to focus on your form and breathing.

FreeStyle Jumping

This part of your workout in many ways defines what makes RopeSport different from traditional jumping rope. Plainly and simply, what you're doing when you FreeStyle is combining jumps and Rope Turns in any order you want for as long as it feels good to you. Maybe you're going in and out of the rope. Maybe you're changing speeds from fast to slow and slow to fast. And maybe you're doing all of these things.

You should incorporate 20 to 60 seconds of FreeStyling at various points throughout your workout. While I give specific ideas about when you should FreeStyle in the sections of this book where I suggest specific workouts (chapters 12, 15, 18), you should feel free to FreeStyle whenever the feeling moves you. Regardless of your skill level, at the beginning of your workout your FreeStyling should be at a moderate pace with beginning to intermediate jumps. This will give you a chance to get a really good feel for the rope before you consider picking up the pace and letting it all hang out. For example, go in and out of the rope using Figure 8 Entrances, Figure 8 Exits, 2 Foot Jumps, the Alternating Foot, and the Run. If you're a beginner, just continue to do this type of basic FreeStyling intermittently throughout your workout. If you're an intermediate or advanced jumper, as you're further into your workout I'd suggest picking up the pace and incorporating a wider variety of jumps and rope turns into your FreeStyling.

Cool Down

By the time you finish the cardio portion of your workout your heart rate should definitely be elevated. Maybe you're even ready to drop dead (just kidding!). Therefore, it's important that you spend at least a few minutes to gradually lower your heart rate and cool down. A great way to do this is to execute a variety of Resting Moves at a very slow pace. Use any combination of Figure 8s, 2 Turns to Each Side, or Step Touches. This is an especially important time to connect with your breathing.

Water Break

Take a water break for a few minutes (but no longer) in order to hydrate yourself. If you sweat a lot during your workout, it's even more important that you replenish your body with fluids. Drinking a lot of water before, during, and after your workout will also help you to recover faster. I suggest that you walk around during this break in order to keep your muscles warm.

Strength, Muscle Conditioning, and Toning

I love to follow the cardio portion of my workout with a few minutes of muscle conditioning and toning. While you continue to burn fat during this part of your workout, you'll also be shaping all the major muscle groups of your upper and lower body. If you've been working hard until now, you're very possibly feeling tired. You're almost done, so try to hang in there for just a few more minutes. Before you begin, check in with your breathing and refocus your energy in order to get the most from these exercises.

Hurray, you're almost done!

Stretch and Flexibility

After your workout is actually the best time to stretch and improve your flexibility. The reason is that your muscles are really warm after you've trained, enabling you to go deeper into most stretches. A good analogy is a rubber band—the warmer it is, the more you can stretch it. The same is true for your muscles.

You did it.

Chapter 8

RopeSport Fundamentals

The following five techniques will serve as the foundation for all the jumps and moves that follow. After learning these fundamentals, you will have the necessary building blocks to begin a safe, effective workout program.

Figure 8

The Figure 8 is the most frequently used Rope Turn and Resting Move and the move I begin my classes with. Start with your feet shoulder-width apart so you have a good base to work from. Grip each handle individually and push the handles together. Begin to cross the rope from one side of your body to the other in what we call a Figure 8 motion. You can also think of it as making a big X. The rope should be grazing or just missing the ground on each side, and if the rope is slapping the ground you should adjust the level of your hands. Your elbows are in and next to your torso, not extended away from your body. Try to remain loose and relaxed in your upper body

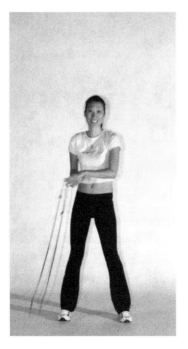

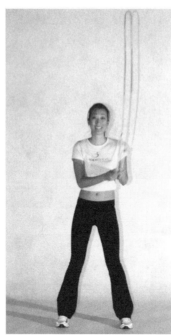

and don't tighten up. *Be sure the handles stay together and don't let them separate*; it's much harder to control the rope if your hands come apart. The verbal cue I use when teaching the Figure 8 is "*turn turn turn turn*" or "*cross cross cross cross.*" Turn the rope slowly at first. When you get more comfortable with the motion, try turning the rope a little faster, gradually increasing speed until you're turning it to the beat of the music. Remind yourself to keep your elbows in, stay loose and relaxed, and be sure to keep the handles together. It's

cross / cross / cross / cross or
it's turn / turn / turn / turn.

Alternating Foot (also known as the Figure 8 Bouncing)

Begin by doing the Figure 8 with your feet stationary. Whenever you're ready, bring your feet closer together and begin to bounce. Use both hands while you continue to cross the rope from one side of your body to the other in an X, just like you did with the stationary Figure 8—what's different is the footwork. Basically, your feet are taking a little hop from one side to the other. It's

hop right / hop left / hop right / hop left /
hop right / hop left / hop right / hop left.

Now this move can feel awkward at first and takes a little getting used to, but just be patient and soon it'll feel really comfortable. A great way to learn the Figure 8 Bouncing is to do the footwork without the rope first, then add the rope whenever you're ready.

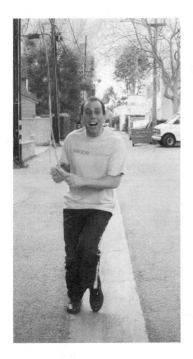
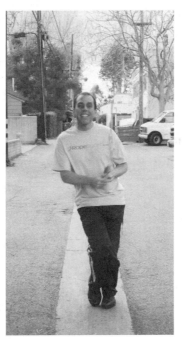

You should keep a couple of important pointers in mind while you're doing the Figure 8 Bouncing. First, try to keep the rope turning at the same speed while you continue to bounce and *don't let the rope slow down*, something that can really throw off your timing and that's a very common tendency when learning this move. It's *turn turn turn turn* or *cross cross cross cross* to the beat of the music (music is a huge help here, too!). Make sure the handles stay together and don't let them separate.

It's important to know that everyone does the Figure 8 Bouncing a little differently with their own individual flavor. We all have our own different groove or way that we move naturally, and incorporating that into your workout is an integral part of the RopeSport style of jumping. Imagine that the rope is your dance partner and you're just dancing with your rope.

Figure 8 Entrance

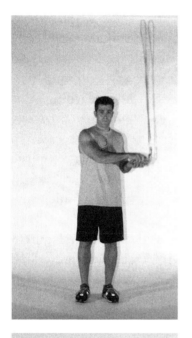

The Figure 8 Entrance is the technique you use to transition from the Figure 8 Rope Turn, where the rope is turning to the side of your body, to actually jumping through the rope.

Stationary

Start by doing the Figure 8 Rope Turn with your feet on the ground and close together. When the rope passes over your head, begin to separate the handles. This will create an opening in the rope, allowing you to enter the rope and begin jumping through it.

Make sure you keep the handles together until the rope passes over your head; if you separate them too soon it's a lot harder to enter the rope cleanly. Keep practicing until you make the entrance smooth and effortless. And you want to practice entering from both sides of your body, right and left.

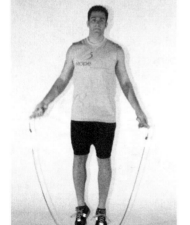

Bouncing

The next step is to execute the Figure 8 Entrance with your feet bouncing. This one might take a few tries, but it's a very important move that you'll pick up with a little practice.

Just like with the stationary entrance, separate the handles as the rope passes over your head (not before), enter the rope, and begin jumping. If you're having trouble entering the rope cleanly, there's a good chance that it's because you're allowing the rope to slow down immediately before you enter, so concentrate on maintaining a steady tempo. And be sure to practice entering from both sides of your body, right and left.

2 Foot Jump

It is extremely important to develop a solid, energy-efficient 2 Foot Jump. It is *the* essential building block for all other jumps that follow, so let's break it down step by step.

A critical component of the 2 Foot Jump is the position of your arms and how you're turning the rope. You should be using some wrist and some forearm to turn the rope. Think of making small circles or a cranking motion. Be sure to use a combination of both wrist and forearm when turning the rope. In fact, one of the most common mistakes I've seen with beginning jumpers is that they turn the rope with their arms extending way away from their torso, using only their wrists and very little forearm. This causes the shoulders to do most of the work and, as a result, an unnecessary expenditure of energy due to improper jumping technique.

Something else that can cause the arms to extend away from your torso and into an incorrect jumping position is using a rope that's too long. It forces your arms to

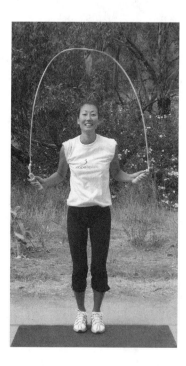
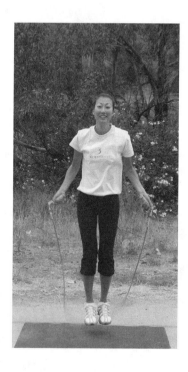

compensate for the improper length, while a rope that's sized properly allows the arms to remain in a natural, relaxed position. Again, you want to try to keep your elbows right by your torso and make sure that your forearms are angled toward the front and not extended way out to your sides. If your arms are in the correct position and you're turning the rope with a balance of wrist and forearm, the result is a relaxed, energy-efficient rotation action. We refer to it as having a smooth stroke, and it's something you should focus on from your very first workout.

Another important element of proper jumping technique is only jumping a few inches off the ground, just enough room to let the rope pass under your feet. Remember that jumping rope is about timing, not how high you jump. Another common mistake for beginning jumpers is that they jump far too high off the ground, causing them to use a lot of excess energy and to land with way too much impact. When you're jumping with proper form there is very little impact, much less than in many other aerobic activities and far less than running. As a beginning jumper, constantly remind yourself to land softly. Some mental imagery I've found helpful is to imagine you're jumping on a glass floor; if you land too hard, you break the floor.

Try to keep your shoulders down and relaxed, not up

and tight. Your knees should remain soft and act like shock absorbers. You're pushing up off the balls of your feet, and your heels are just tapping the ground. Your hands should stay level with your hips; don't let them raise or the rope will catch on your feet. This is a common error when you're learning a new jump; while your body goes up, your hands should stay down.

One last thing we see with a lot of beginning jumpers is that they'll take an extra little jump or what we call the Bunny Hop. The basic rule of thumb when you're starting out is to take one jump per revolution of the rope, not two (the exception to this rule is with more advanced jumps like Doubles where the rope rotates two times per jump). There's nothing inherently wrong with the Bunny Hop. In fact, it's very gentle on the body. However, it will limit your ability to execute a lot of different jumps and if possible should be avoided. Usually the Bunny Hop is caused by turning the rope too slowly, forcing you to take an extra jump while you're waiting for the rope to come around. A simple correction is to *turn the rope faster*. Something else that can help fix the Bunny Hop is to try jumping to the beat of the music.

Figure 8 Exit

The Figure 8 Exit is how you transition from jumping through the rope to turning the rope to the side of your body. In other words, it's how you exit the rope and begin to do Rope Turns.

In a nutshell, with the Figure 8 Exit you reverse what you did for the Figure 8 Entrance—that is, as you're jumping through the rope and it passes over your head, bring one handle over until it meets the other handle on the side of your body. At this point your hands are together and you transition to Rope Turns. Just like with the Figure 8 Entrance, practice exiting to both sides of your body, right and left. Try making the exit smooth and relaxed and continue to turn the rope at the same tempo without missing a beat.

Chapter 9

Rope Turns

Rope Turns are defined as any time you're turning the rope to the side of your body and not jumping through the rope. When done at a slow to moderate pace, they allow you to recover and are called Resting Moves, something that's essential for jumpers of all skill levels, especially beginners. When done at a fast tempo, they allow you to get a fat-blasting workout without even jumping through the rope. Equally as important, they add variety to your workout. They are an integral part of the RopeSport jumping philosophy and training method.

Basic Rope Turns and Resting Moves

Figure 8

See chapter 8, "RopeSport Fundamentals."

2 Turns to Each Side

In addition to the Figure 8, one of the most frequently used Rope Turns and Resting Moves is the 2 Turns to Each Side. With your feet shoulder-width apart, push the

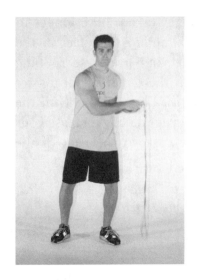

handles together and turn the rope to the side of your body with the Figure 8 Rope Turn in an X motion. Whenever you're ready, execute one additional Rope Turn on each side of your body with the rope at 12 and 6 o'clock. *It's two rotations on your right side, then two rotations on your left side; two rotations on your right side, then two rotations on your left side.* And once you get a feel for it, try speeding it up a little and getting more aggressive, gradually working toward turning the rope to the beat of the music. Just like with the Figure 8, make sure you keep the handles together and stay loose and relaxed; the rope should be just grazing the ground. Keep your elbows in by your torso and not extended away from your torso. It's

cross / turn / cross / turn /
cross / turn / cross / turn.

2 Turns Step Touch

The 2 Turns Step Touch is a progression from the 2 Turns to Each Side.

Start with the 2 Turns to Each Side with your feet stationary and about shoulder-width apart. As you execute

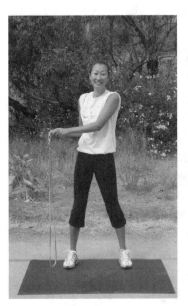
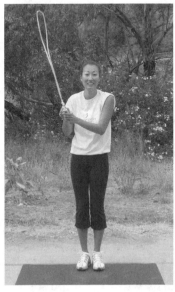

the second rotation of the rope on your right side, your left foot takes a step to the right and touches next to your right foot. At the same time the rope crosses in front of you from right to left, take a step to the side with your left foot so your feet are shoulder-width apart again. As the rope rotates a second time on your left, take a step left with your right foot and touch next to your left foot. Continue to repeat.

The 2 Turns Step Touch might take a little longer to learn because you're using your hands and feet at the same time, kind of like patting your head and rubbing your stomach, but just hang in there and you'll master it in a few practice sessions. Just like you did with the Figure 8 and 2 Turns to Each Side, gradually increase your speed until you're turning the rope to the beat of the music. It's

step / touch / step / touch /
step / touch / step / touch.

Figure 8 High and Low

Whether jumping through the rope or executing Rope Turns, you usually want the rope just grazing the ground. However, you can also raise your hands so you're executing the Figure 8 with the rope crossing above your head. It's the perfect time to add your own groove and personal style. I suggest alternating from low to high and vice versa.

Backward

Just like jumping backward, virtually every Rope Turn and Resting Move can and should be done backward! It is no harder than doing them forward. And don't argue with me—*just do it!*

Intermediate Rope Turns

One-Hand Variation

When you're first learning Rope Turns I suggest using two hands to execute the moves. It's easier to control the rope that way. However, as soon as your skill level progresses you should put both grips in one hand and execute many of the same Rope Turns using one hand only. Start with the Figure 8 Stationary and Figure 8 Bouncing, 2 Turns to Each Side, and 2 Turns Step Touch. Many intermediate and advanced jumpers prefer doing a majority of Rope Turns with one hand instead of two.

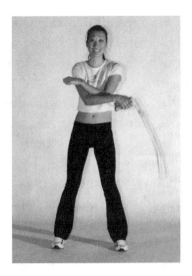 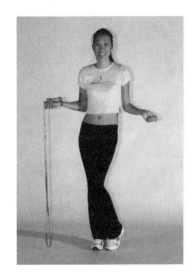

Funky Step Touch

The Funky Step Touch (aka the Lunge) is a modification of the 2 Turns Step Touch. The rotation motion of the rope is exactly the same. Instead of stepping from side to side, however, you're going to add a bounce to your step while simultaneously turning your shoulders so they're facing whatever direction you're moving toward. It's time to get a little funky.

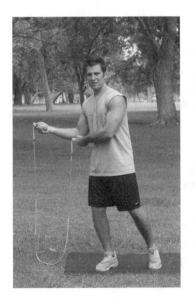 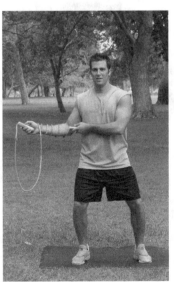

Arm Wrap

The Arm Wrap is primarily a finesse move. Start by doing a Figure 8 Rope Turn. As the rope crosses to your right side, extend your right arm outward and bring your left hand over until the grip is positioned next to the elbow of your right arm. Next, rotate the wrist of your right hand in a forward motion so the rope wraps around your right forearm. After the rope is wrapped all the way around your right forearm, cross both arms over to the left side of your torso (they should now be mirroring the position they were in on the right). In order to complete the Arm Wrap, rotate your right wrist in a backward motion and the rope will unwrap from your right forearm.

Hand over Hand

Hand over Hand is similar to the 2 Turns to Each Side. Instead of keeping the handles together, however, as you cross to one side you separate the handles with the hand that's positioned on top leading for the first rotation of the rope. For the second rotation of the rope, the hands come back together. Then repeat on the other side.

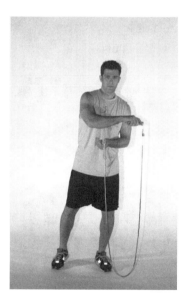
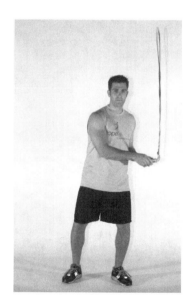

Advanced Rope Turns

3 Turns to Each Side

The 3 Turns to Each Side Rope Turn is a progression from the 2 Turns to Each Side. As the name suggests, you execute one additional rotation of the rope to each side of your body. Start slowly and gradually increase your speed. Try to make small, tight circles with your wrists. If you reach the point at which you're doing the 3 Turns to Each

Side to the tempo of the music, the rope will be flying. It's almost like a rapid-fire staccato. It's

one two three / one two three / one two three /
one two three / one two three / one two three /
one two three / one two three.

Butterfly

The Butterfly might take some time to learn, but it looks supercool and will impress the heck out of whoever's watching. Start with the Figure 8 Rope Turn with both hands together. As the rope reaches your right side, begin to separate your hands, with your left hand sweeping over your head from right to left and your right hand passing behind you in the same direction (right to left). When your right hand reaches your left side, bring it up and over until your right and left hands come together. To complete the Butterfly, execute one more rope rotation on your left side. The Butterfly can be done on either side, left or right.

Behind the Back

Start with a one-hand Figure 8 using your right hand. Whenever you're ready, instead of crossing the rope in front, bring it behind your torso and pass both handles from your right to left hand.

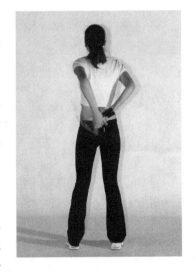

Body Wrap

Start the Body Wrap with a Figure 8 Rope Turn with both hands together. Separate the handles so one hand is by your waist while the other hand is positioned above your head. Rotate the hand that's above your head and the rope will wrap around your body. In order to unwrap the rope, rotate the hand that's above your head in the opposite direction.

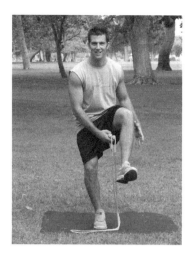

Under the Leg Pass

Start the Under the Leg Pass with a one-hand Figure 8 with the grips in your right hand. On the downward swing of the rope, lift your left leg while you bring your right hand under and pass the grips from your right to left hand.

Changing Directions

As you become a more proficient jumper, you want to frequently transition from jumping forward to backward and vice versa. There are a few different ways to accomplish this.

Arm Wrap

In addition to being an Intermediate Rope Turn, you can also use Arm Wraps to change directions from forward to backward. As the rope unwraps from your forearm to complete the Arm Wrap (see Intermediate Rope Turns), you can easily transition to backward Rope Turns, and from there to backward jumping.

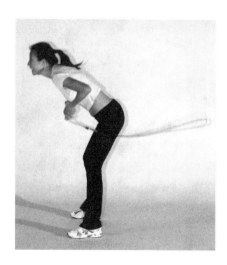

Through the Legs

Start with the 2 Foot Jump with the rope rotating forward. Whenever you're ready, stop jumping, and with your feet stationary and your body bent slightly forward, slow the rope down and bring it between your legs. After the rope comes to a stop, bring your arms back through your legs and in front of your body so the rope is rotating backward. Immediately transition into a Backward Figure 8 Rope Turn. Use a Backward Figure 8 Entrance to enter the rope into a Backward 2 Foot Jump.

Heel Catch

The Heel Catch is another way to change directions. While jumping backward, simply stop jumping so your

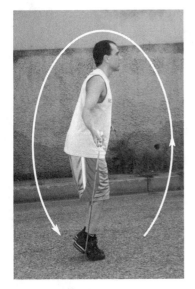

feet are stationary and you're on the balls of your feet with your heels raised. As the rope comes around, it will catch under your feet and come to a complete stop. At that point you can either stop completely and walk away looking really cool or, if you want to keep jumping, bring your arms forward and enter the rope into a Forward 2 Foot Jump.

Toe Catch with a Kick

Begin with a Forward Figure 8 Rope Turn. Extend your right foot out in front of you and plant your right heel into the ground. As the rope comes around, it will catch under your right foot (and if you're done for the day this is another way to stop the rope completely and exit). After it stops under your foot, pull the handles back toward you so all the slack is out and the rope is tight against your right heel. Bring your right foot in toward you, then kick out, and the rope will begin rotating backward, at which time you'll transition into a Backward Figure 8 Rope Turn. Whenever you're ready, use a Backward Figure 8 Entrance to enter the rope and begin jumping backward with a 2 Foot Jump.

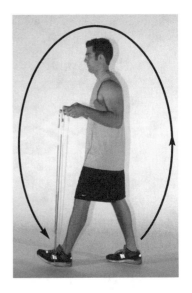

Changing direction from backward to forward and vice versa is an integral part of the RopeSport style of jumping. As I emphasized earlier, jumping backward is something most people don't focus on, to their own detriment. There simply is no good reason for you not to be jumping backward each and every workout.

Part II

JUMP IN
Exercises That
Take You through
Beginning,
Intermediate,
Advanced, and
Extreme Moves
and Workouts

Chapter 10

Basic Jumps

In this section I'll focus on a variety of Basic Jumps, many of which you can master in just a few workouts. It's very important to jump with proper form and technique when executing these moves. As with many other sports and exercises, you always need to focus on the fundamentals and go back to the basics. Finally, remember that you can use the Three-Step Breakdown to learn any of these jumps.

Wherever appropriate, I've also included the verbal cues that I use in my group exercise classes *in italics*. Over the years I've found it helpful to actually say these verbal cues out loud when learning a new jump. It's the mind-body connection in action.

By the end of this section I hope you'll have a sense of the wide variety of jumps that you can incorporate into your RopeSport workout, even as a beginning jumper. And because of this variety, you'll be able to constantly challenge yourself and stay motivated. Just be patient, and in a few workouts you'll be well on your way.

Front/Back

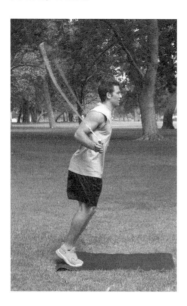

The first Basic Jump you're going to learn is the Front/Back, and it's done by doing exactly that—jumping to the front and then to the back. It's fun, easy, and great for improving your core stability. Start center with your feet in the 2-Foot-Jump position. On the first rotation of the rope you jump forward 6 to 12 inches; on the next rotation of the rope you jump back 6 to 12 inches. Continue to repeat. It's

front / back / front / back /
front / back / front / back.

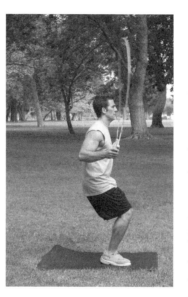

The turning motion of the rope is exactly the same as it is for the 2 Foot Jump; the only thing that's different is the footwork. Your elbows are by your torso, and your forearms are angled forward. Turn the rope with some wrist and forearm, making small circles. Only jump a few inches off the ground, just enough to let the rope pass under your feet. Try to land softly with very little impact. Shoulders are down and relaxed. You're jumping to the beat of the music and not letting the rope slow down or speed up. You're pushing off the balls of your feet and your legs are acting as shock absorbers. Keep it nice and safe and controlled.

Slalom

The slalom is done by jumping from one side to the other side. It'll do wonders for your balance and lateral movement. Start center with your feet in the 2-Foot-Jump position. On the first rotation of the rope, jump to the right 6 to 12 inches. On the next rotation of the rope, jump to the left 6 to 12 inches. Continue to repeat. It's

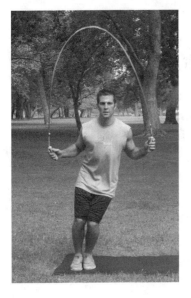

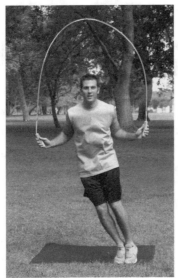

*right / left / right / left /
right / left / right / left.*

It's a fun and easy jump that you'll master with a little practice.

Straddle

The footwork for the Straddle is exactly like it is for a jumping jack. Start center with your feet in the 2-Foot-Jump position. On the first rotation of the rope, your feet separate and move out to the sides. On the next rotation of the rope, bring both feet back in to center position where they were for the 2 Foot Jump. Continue to repeat. It's

*out / center /out /center /
out /center /out / center.*

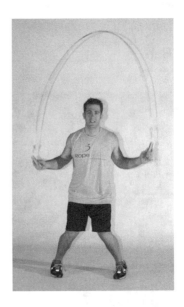

Lunge

The Lunge (or Scissor) targets the quadriceps, hamstrings, and glutes, like a minilunge. It's done by separating your feet and scissoring them.

Start center with your feet in the 2-Foot-Jump position. On the first rotation of the rope, separate your feet with your right foot moving forward in front of your torso and

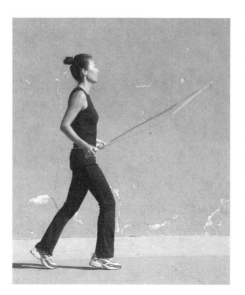

your left foot behind. On the next rotation of the rope, reverse the position of your feet with your left foot forward and your right foot behind you. Continue to repeat.

Remind yourself that the position of your arms and the turning motion of the rope is exactly the same as in the 2 Foot Jump. Elbows in, turn with some wrist and arm, land softly, and keep the tempo the same. The only thing that changes is the position of your feet.

What are you waiting for? Give it a shot! It's

scissor / scissor / scissor / scissor /
or *lunge / lunge / lunge / lunge.*

Run

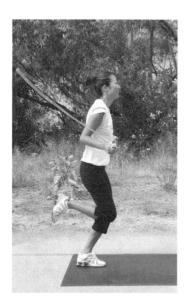

The name says it all. You're simply running through the rope. And because the running motion is one you're familiar with, something you've done since you were a kid, this one's a cinch. Start center with your feet in the 2-Foot-Jump position and begin to run. Continue to repeat. It's

run / run / run / run / run / run / run / run.

While a lot of workouts, including aerobics, spinning, and running, focus primarily on the lower body, a unique advantage of jumping rope is that due to the constant turning motion of the rope, your upper body also gets a fantastic workout. And because you're utilizing *all* the major muscle groups of your body, jumping rope is a phenomenal cardiovascular exercise that will help you burn an incredible amount of fat—up to a thousand calories an hour! It's also one of the best exercises for getting rid of cellulite and developing shapely calves and ankles. Another benefit of jumping rope is that because it is a weight-bearing activity, it helps build stronger bones and reduce any chance of developing osteoporosis, something that's especially important to a lot of women.

Toe In/Toe Out

The Toe In/Toe Out, affectionately known as the Duck, is a fun move that you'll learn quickly. Start center with your feet in the 2-Foot-Jump position. On the first rotation of the rope, turn your feet in so you're pigeon-toed. On the second rotation of the rope, turn your feet so they're facing out. Continue to repeat. It's

in / out / in / out / in / out / in / out.
("Quack quack quack quack.")

Boxer Shuffle

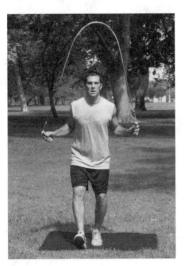

This next jump is popular with a lot of boxers, so I named it the Boxer Shuffle. You're just digging your heels in, alternating one foot and then the other. Start center with your feet in the 2-Foot-Jump position. On the first rotation of the rope, your right heel moves forward and digs into the ground while your left foot stays in center position. On the next rotation of the rope, move your left foot forward and dig with your left heel while your right foot stays in center position. Continue to repeat. It's

heel / heel / heel / heel or *dig / dig / dig / dig.*

Make sure that your feet aren't kicking in the air, a common error. Rather, whatever foot is in the forward position, the heel of that foot actually touches the ground.

Speaking of boxers, arguably the most well-conditioned athletes in the world, who use jumping rope as an indispensable part of their training routines, another great benefit of jumping rope is that it will maximize all your athletic skills. You'll see major improvement in your speed and power development, timing, footwork, agility, and coordination. These are skills that contribute greatly to athletic prowess and are essential to almost any sport you can think of. That's why so many athletes, coaches, and fitness professionals I've worked with swear by the Rope-Sport training method and consider it a phenomenal cross-training workout.

Alternating Foot

The Alternating Foot is another jump you see boxers do. The foot movement is identical to the Bouncing Figure 8 Rope Turn. The difference is that now you're executing it while jumping through the rope. The Alternating Foot might take a little more time to learn than some of the other Basic Jumps. However, it's the most energy-efficient jump you can do, and you should work on it right from the start. In other words, it requires less expenditure of energy per revolution than any other jump. When you're

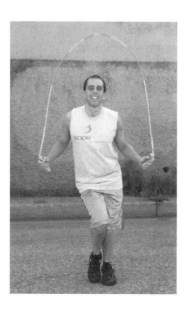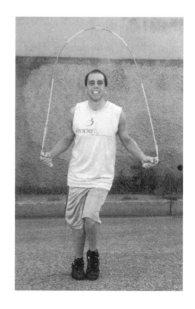

doing the Alternate Foot with proper form, you can even catch your breath while you continue to jump!

Start center with the 2 Foot Jump. On the first rotation of the rope, shift your weight to the right while taking a little hop to your right side. As your right foot lands, your left heel is raised and you're on the ball of your left foot. On the second rotation of the rope you reverse position by shifting your weight to your left and taking a small hop; your left foot is down on the ground while your right heel is raised and you're on the ball of your right foot. Start slowly at first and then increase your speed. Continue to repeat. It's

hop left / hop right / hop left / hop right / hop left / hop right / hop left / hop right.

When you're executing the Alternating Foot with proper form and technique, it requires so little energy that you should be able to breathe normally and carry on a conversation with someone while you continue to jump. It's just a walk in the park.

If you're having trouble mastering any new jump, practice it for a few minutes each workout, then move on to a different jump. Come back to it later or wait until your next workout to try it again. I guarantee you that if you approach your workout this way, you'll learn most of the Basic Jumps in just a few short practice sessions. Try not to get frustrated. Sometimes learning a new jump, the Alternating Foot, for example, is just like learning to ride a bike. It can take a few tries, but just be patient and all of a sudden you'll be executing the jump with no problem at all.

Alternating Knee Up

As with a number of jumps you can use in your RopeSport workout, the Alternating Knee Up was taken right out of aerobics class. Start center with the 2 Foot Jump. On the first rotation of the rope, raise your right knee up in front while your left foot stays in center position and continues to bounce. On the second rotation of the rope, your right

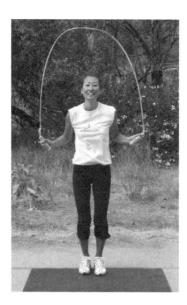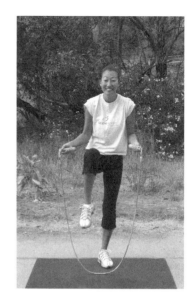

foot comes back to center and you take one jump with both feet. On the third rotation of the rope, your left knee raises while you bounce one time on your right foot. To complete the move, your left foot comes back to center and you take one jump on both feet. Continue to repeat. It's

right knee up / center / left knee up /
center / right knee up / center / left knee up /
center / right knee up / center / left knee up.

The raising of each leg independently does wonders for shaping your hips and butt. Be careful that you're not doing a Run here, a mistake I see fairly often. The difference is that with the Alternating Knee Up you're taking a bounce in the center with both feet between each knee coming up.

Backward 2 Foot Jump

Many times I've seen people who are great jumpers but for some inexplicable reason have never practiced jumping backward. When I tell them they should also be jumping backward they get a surprised look on their face. Finally, when they stubbornly agree to give it a try, they look like they're starting over. Well, let me tell you something that

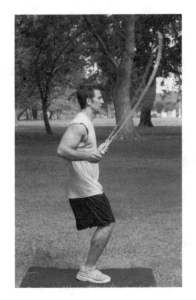

you absolutely, positively need to know about jumping backward—it is no more difficult than jumping forward! You just have to practice.

The *only* difference between jumping backward and jumping forward is that your wrists are rotating in the opposite direction—that is, backward. Keep the exact same pointers in mind as you did with the Forward 2 Foot Jump. You're only jumping a few inches off the ground and landing softly. Elbows are in and you're turning the rope with some wrist and forearm cranking motion. Shoulders are down and relaxed. You're jumping to the beat of the music and not letting the rope slow down or speed up. You're pushing off the balls of your feet and your legs are acting as shock absorbers.

And while jumping backward is great for all your major muscle groups, it's killer on your biceps. By jumping backward you're also adding variety to your workout by literally doubling the jumps you can do. Virtually all the Rope Turns and Basic Jumps can and should be done backward. Double the jumps means double the fun.

Crosses

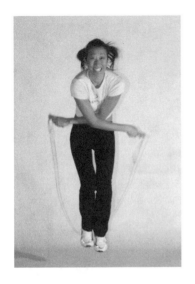

This jump, the Cross, is probably the one you remember from your local school playground. Are you ready to feel like a kid again?!

Start center with the 2 Foot Jump. When the rope passes over your head, cross your arms in front of you. With your arms in the crossed position, jump through the rope. When the rope passes under your feet and is behind you, uncross your arms. Continue to repeat. It's

*cross / uncross / cross / uncross /
cross / uncross / cross / uncross.*

There are a few specific pointers to the Cross that I want to review with you. Because it's the only Basic Jump where the hands move into a totally different position (crossed instead of to the side of your torso), you might need a little more practice before you master it. So be patient, and you'll have it down before you know it.

First, make sure that when your hands are in the crossed position they extend as far past your torso as possible. This will create a nice arc and give you more space to jump through. If you don't extend your arms far enough while they're in the crossed position, the opening won't be big enough to get your body through.

Second, your hands stay level with your hips while executing the Cross. If your hands raise up, the rope will catch on your legs. If you lower your hands the rope will hit the ground far too hard, interrupting the rotation and throwing off your timing. Third, make sure your hands hug your hips, and don't let them extend forward away from your body. Finally, don't change the speed of your rotation.

Keep it nice and relaxed. At first try doing one Cross at a time. Then put a few together consecutively. Go for it!

Chapter 11

Basic Jump Combinations

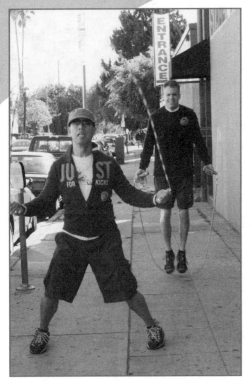

Now that you've mastered a variety of individual jumps, it's time to put them together into different combinations. By doing so you'll continue to challenge yourself, stay motivated, and add an element of creativity to your workout. You'll also make your jump rope workout fun and more effective!

What follows are some suggestions for Basic Jump Combinations. These choreographed routines are similar to what you find in other group exercise classes, including step and aerobics.

All jump combinations are written out in sets of eight counts (shown in *italics* below each jump). You can make combinations longer by either repeating each individual jump for an additional eight counts or repeating the entire combination. I recommend you start off slowly, making sure to utilize Resting Moves between sets. Soon you'll be combining the combinations!

Just as with the jumps, you can always begin by trying the combinations without the rope to get a feel for the footwork. Once you get going, you'll see how much fun putting the different jumps together can be!

All these jumps are described in detail in chapter 10, "Basic Jumps."

Basic Jump Combination 1

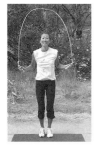 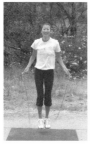

2 Foot Jump

jump / jump / jump / jump /
jump / jump / jump / jump

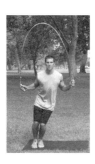 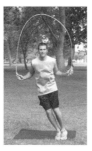

Slalom

right / left / right / left / right / left / right / left

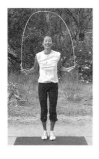 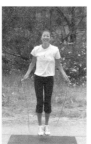

2 Foot Jump

jump / jump / jump / jump /
jump / jump / jump / jump

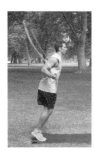 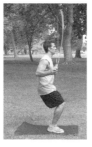

Front/Back

front / back / front / back / front / back / front / back

Basic Jump Combination 2

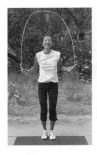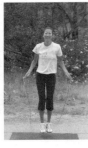

2 Foot Jump

jump / jump / jump / jump /
jump / jump / jump / jump

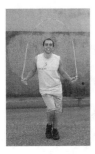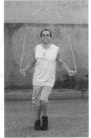

Alternating Foot

hop right / hop left / hop right / hop left /
hop right / hop left / hop right / hop left

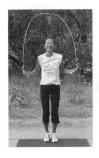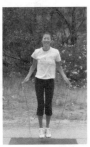

2 Foot Jump

jump / jump / jump / jump /
jump / jump / jump / jump

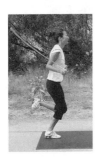

Run

run right / run left / run right / run left /
run right / run left / run right / run left

Basic Jump Combination 3

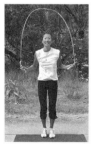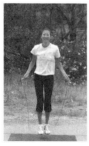

2 Foot Jump

jump / jump / jump / jump /
jump / jump / jump / jump

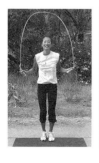

Lunge

lunge right / lunge left / lunge right / lunge left /
lunge right / lunge left / lunge right / lunge left

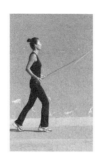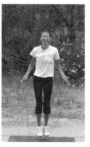

2 Foot Jump

jump / jump / jump / jump /
jump / jump / jump / jump

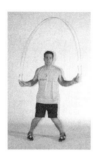

Straddle

out / center / out / center / out / center / out / center

Basic Jump Combination 4

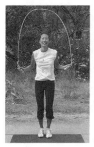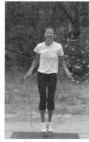

2 Foot Jump

jump / jump / jump / jump /
jump / jump / jump / jump

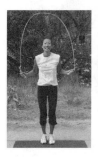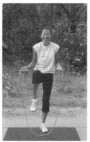

Alternating Knee Up

right knee up / center / left knee up / center /
right knee up / center / left knee up / center

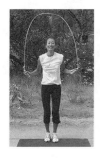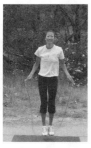

2 Foot Jump

jump / jump / jump / jump /
jump / jump / jump / jump

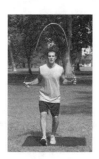

Boxer Shuffle

dig right / dig left / dig right / dig left /
dig right / dig left / dig right / dig left

Basic Jump Combination 5

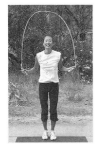 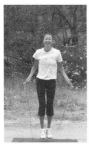

2 Foot Jump

jump / jump / jump / jump /
jump / jump / jump / jump

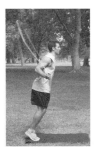 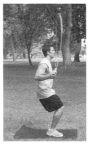

Front/Back

front / back / front / back /
front / back / front / back

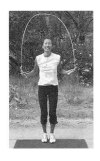 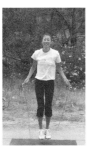

2 Foot Jump

jump / jump / jump / jump /
jump / jump / jump / jump

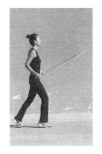

Lunge

lunge right / lunge left / lunge right / lunge left /
lunge right / lunge left / lunge right / lunge left

Basic Jump Combination 6

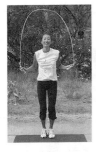 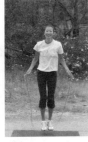

2 Foot Jump

jump / jump / jump / jump /
jump / jump / jump / jump

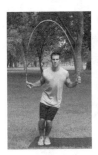 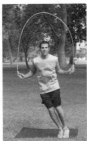

Slalom

right / left / right / left /
right / left / right / left

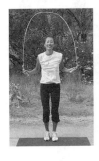 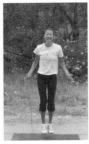

2 Foot Jump

jump / jump / jump / jump /
jump / jump / jump / jump

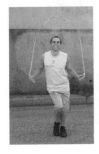 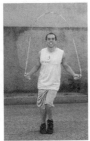

Alternating Foot

hop right / hop left / hop right / hop left /
hop right / hop left / hop right / hop left

Basic Jump Combination 7

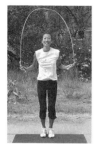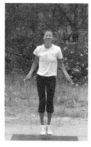

2 Foot Jump

jump / jump / jump / jump /
jump / jump / jump / jump

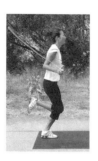

Run

run right / run left / run right / run left /
run right / run left / run right / run left

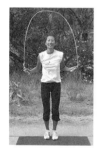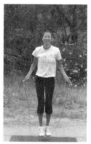

2 Foot Jump

jump / jump / jump / jump /
jump / jump / jump / jump

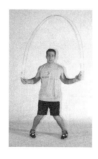

Straddle

out / center / out / center /
out / center / out / center

Basic Jump Combination 8

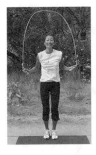 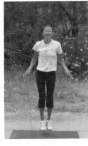

2 Foot Jump

jump / jump / jump / jump /
jump / jump / jump / jump

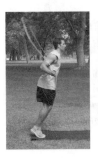 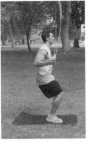

Front/Back

front / back / front / back /
front / back / front / back

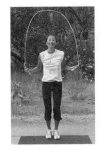 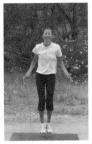

2 Foot Jump

jump / jump / jump / jump /
jump / jump / jump / jump

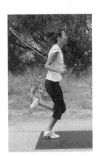

Run

run right / run left / run right / run left /
run right / run left / run right / run left

Basic Jump Combination 9

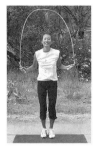 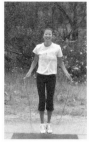

2 Foot Jump

*jump / jump / jump / jump /
jump / jump / jump / jump*

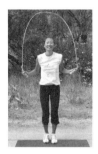 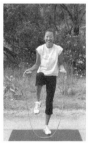

Alternating Knee Up

*right knee up / center / left knee up / center /
right knee up / center / left knee up / center*

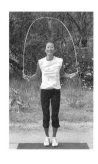 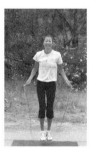

2 Foot Jump

*jump / jump / jump / jump /
jump / jump / jump / jump*

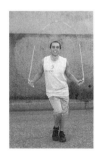 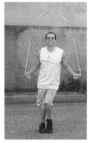

Alternating Foot

*hop right / hop left / hop right / hop left /
hop right / hop left / hop right / hop left*

Basic Jump Combination 10

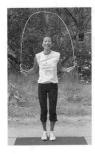 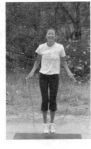

2 Foot Jump

jump / jump / jump / jump /
jump / jump / jump / jump

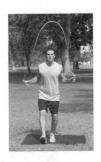

Boxer Shuffle

dig right / dig left / dig right / dig left /
dig right / dig left / dig right / dig left

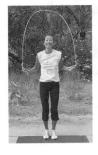 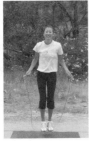

2 Foot Jump

jump / jump / jump / jump /
jump / jump / jump / jump

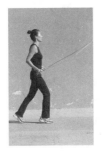

Lunge

lunge right / lunge left / lunge right / lunge left /
lunge right / lunge left / lunge right / lunge left

Basic Jump Combination Bonus #1: Vertical Movement

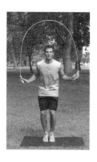

2 Foot Jump, in place

jump / jump / jump / jump / jump / jump / jump / jump

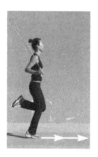

Run, traveling forward

run right / run left / run right / run left / run right / run left / run right / run left

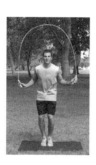

2 Foot Jump, in place

jump / jump / jump / jump / jump / jump / jump / jump

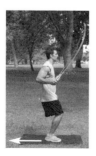

2 Foot Jump, traveling backward

jump back / jump back / jump back / jump back / jump back / jump back / jump back / jump back

Basic Jump Combination Bonus #2: Increased Difficulty

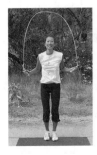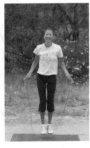

2 Foot Jump

jump / jump / jump / jump /
jump / jump / jump / jump

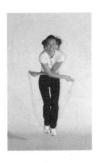

Cross

cross / uncross / cross / uncross /
cross / uncross / cross / uncross

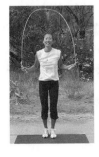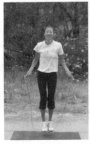

2 Foot Jump

jump / jump / jump / jump /
jump / jump / jump / jump

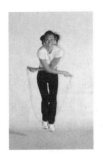

Cross

cross / uncross / cross / uncross /
cross / uncross / cross / uncross

Chapter 12

Basic RopeSport Workouts

(120–125 beats per minute; 15–20 minutes)

Use the following workouts on a weekly rotation. They should last you about a month. As your skill level improves, feel free to mix and match to fit your own unique style. Please note that the Basic Workout Grid on page 106 is meant to be used as a quick reference guide. The grid does not include Resting Moves between the jump sections or specific moves for the Stretches or Cooldowns. Please refer to the workout section below for a detailed list of the Stretches, Resting Moves, and Cooldowns.

Workout 1

Warm-up

- FreeStyle Rope Turns (1 minute)
- Figure 8 (4 × 8 counts)
- 2 Turns to Each Side (4 × 8 counts)
- Figure 8 (4 × 8 counts)
- Figure 8 Bouncing (4 × 8 counts)
- 2 Foot Jump (2 × 8 counts)
- Figure 8 (2 × 8 counts)

- Figure 8 Bouncing (2 × 8 counts)
- 2 Foot Jump (2 × 8 counts)
- FreeStyle Jumping (20 seconds)
- Out of the rope
- Recover with Resting Moves (20 seconds)
- Figure 8, right hand (8 counts)
- Figure 8, left hand (8 counts)

Warm-up Stretch (No Rope)

- Inhale 4 counts/exhale 4 counts
  (2 repetitions)
- Neck: head rotation (8 repetitions)
- Neck: head rolls (8 repetitions)
- Shoulders: shoulder circles, front and
  back (8 repetitions each direction)
- Triceps: arms across the body, right and
  left (holding 10 counts each side)
- Chest: hands clasped behind the back
  (holding 10 counts)
- Back: flex and extend (8 repetitions)
- Side and back: waist bend, right and left
  (holding 10 counts each side)
- Hamstrings: standing stretch, right and
  left (holding 10 counts each side)
- Groin and hips: runner's stretch, right
  and left (holding 10 counts each side)
- Hips and lower back: hip circles, right
  and left (8 repetitions each side)
- Ankles, feet, calves, and shins: roll front
  and back (8 repetitions)
- Calves: calf stretch, right and left (holding
  10 counts each side)
- Shins: toe taps, right and left (16 repetitions each side)
- Ankles and feet: ankle circles, right and
  left (8 repetitions each side)

Jump 1

- FreeStyle Rope Turns (4 × 8 counts)
- Figure 8 (2 × 8 counts)
- 2 Turns to Each Side (2 × 8 counts)
- 2 Turns Step Touch (2 × 8 counts)
- Figure 8 (2 × 8 counts)
- Figure 8 Bouncing (2 × 8 counts)
- 2 Foot Jump (3 × 8 counts)
- FreeStyle Jumping (20 seconds)
- Out of the rope
- Recover with Resting Moves (30 seconds
  to 1 minute)

Jump 2

- Figure 8 (2 × 8 counts)
- 2 Turns to Each Side (2 × 8 counts)
- 2 Turns Step Touch (2 × 8 counts)
- Figure 8 (2 × 8 counts)
- Figure 8 Bouncing (2 × 8 counts)
- 2 Foot Jump (3 × 8 counts)
- Alternating Foot (3 × 8 counts)
- FreeStyle Jumping (20 seconds)
- Out of the rope
- Recover with Resting Moves (30 seconds
  to 1 minute)

Sprint Jump

- Figure 8 (2 × 8 counts)
- 2 Turns to Each Side (2 × 8 counts)
- 2 Turns Step Touch (2 × 8 counts)
- Figure 8 (2 × 8 counts)
- Figure 8 Bouncing (2 × 8 counts)
- 2 Foot Jump Sprint (20 seconds)
- Out of the rope
- Recover with Resting Moves (30 seconds
  to 1 minute)

Recovery Jump

- Figure 8 (2 × 8 counts)
- 2 Turns to Each Side (2 × 8 counts)
- 2 Turns Step Touch (2 × 8 counts)
- Figure 8 (2 × 8 counts)
- Figure 8 Bouncing (2 × 8 counts)
- 2 Foot Jump (4 × 8 counts)
- Out of the rope
- Recover with Resting Moves (30 seconds to 1 minute)

Combination

- Figure 8 (2 × 8 counts)
- 2 Turns to Each Side (2 × 8 counts)
- 2 Turns Step Touch (2 × 8 counts)
- Figure 8 (2 × 8 counts)
- Figure 8 Bouncing (2 × 8 counts)
- 2 Foot Jump (2 × 8)
- Combination (1 or 2 sets)
  - 2 Foot Jump (8 counts)
  - Alternating Foot (8 counts)
  - 2 Foot Jump (8 counts)
  - Alternating Foot (8 counts)
- Out of the rope
- Recover with Resting Moves (30 seconds to 1 minute)

Long Jump

- Figure 8 (2 × 8 counts)
- 2 Turns to Each Side (2 × 8 counts)
- 2 Turns Step Touch (2 × 8 counts)
- Figure 8 (2 × 8 counts)
- Figure 8 Bouncing (2 × 8 counts)
- 2 Foot Jump (10 × 8 counts)
- FreeStyle Jumping (30 seconds)

- Out of the rope
- Recover with Resting Moves (30 seconds to 1 minute)

Cooldown

- FreeStyle Rope Turns (1 minute)
- Figure 8 (2 × 8 counts)
- 2 Turns to Each Side (4 × 8 counts)
- 2 Turns Step Touch (4 × 8 counts)
- Figure 8 (2 × 8 counts)
- Figure 8, right hand (8 counts)
- Figure 8, left hand (8 counts)

Strength

- Legs and butt (2 to 3 sets)
  - Squats (8 repetitions)
  Be sure to take a short break between squat sets.

Cooldown Stretch, Standing (No Rope)

- Neck: head rolls (8 repetitions)
- Shoulders: shoulder circles, front and back (8 repetitions each direction)
- Triceps: arms cocked behind head, right and left (holding 10 counts each side)
- Chest: hands clasped behind the back (holding 10 counts)
- Side and back: waist bend, right and left (holding 10 counts each side)
- Hamstrings: standing stretch, right and left (holding 10 counts each side)
- Calves: calf stretch, right and left (holding 10 counts each side)
- Ankles and feet: ankle circles, right and left (8 repetitions each side)
- Inhale 4 counts/exhale 4 counts (2 repetitions)

Workout 2

Warm-up

- FreeStyle Rope Turns (1 minute)
- Figure 8 (4 × 8 counts)
- 2 Turns to Each Side (4 × 8 counts)
- Figure 8 (4 × 8 counts)
- Figure 8 Bouncing (4 × 8 counts)
- 2 Foot Jump (2 × 8 counts)
- Figure 8 (2 × 8 counts)
- Figure 8 Bouncing (2 × 8 counts)
- 2 Foot Jump (2 × 8 counts)
- FreeStyle Jumping (20 seconds)
- Out of the rope
- Recover with Resting Moves (20 seconds)
- Figure 8, right hand (8 counts)
- Figure 8, left hand (8 counts)

Warm-up Stretch (No Rope)

- Inhale 4 counts/exhale 4 counts (2 repetitions)
- Neck: head rotation (8 repetitions)
- Neck: head rolls (8 repetitions)
- Shoulders: shoulder circles, front and back (8 repetitions each direction)
- Triceps: arms across the body, right and left (holding 10 counts each side)
- Chest: hands clasped behind the back (holding 10 counts)
- Back: flex and extend (8 repetitions)
- Side and back: waist bend, right and left (holding 10 counts each side)
- Hamstrings: standing stretch, right and left (holding 10 counts each side)
- Groin and hips: runner's stretch, right and left (holding 10 counts each side)
- Hips and lower back: hip circles, right and left (8 repetitions each side)
- Ankles, feet, calves, and shins: roll front and back (8 repetitions)
- Calves: calf stretch, right and left (holding 10 counts each side)
- Shins: toe taps, right and left (16 repetitions each side)
- Ankles and feet: ankle circles, right and left (8 repetitions each side)

Jump 1

- FreeStyle Rope Turns (4 × 8 counts)
- Figure 8 (2 × 8 counts)
- 2 Turns to Each Side (2 × 8 counts)
- 2 Turns Step Touch (2 × 8 counts)
- Figure 8 (2 × 8 counts)
- Figure 8 Bouncing (2 × 8 counts)
- 2 Foot Jump (3 × 8 counts)
- FreeStyle Jumping (20 seconds)
- Out of the rope
- Recover with Resting Moves (30 seconds to 1 minute)

Jump 2

- Figure 8 (2 × 8 counts)
- 2 Turns to Each Side (2 × 8 counts)
- 2 Turns Step Touch (2 × 8 counts)
- Figure 8 (2 × 8 counts)
- Figure 8 Bouncing (2 × 8 counts)
- 2 Foot Jump (3 × 8 counts)
- Run (3 × 8 counts)
- FreeStyle Jumping (20 seconds)
- Out of the rope
- Recover with Resting Moves (30 seconds to 1 minute)

Sprint Jump

- Figure 8 (2 × 8 counts)
- 2 Turns to Each Side (2 × 8 counts)
- 2 Turns Step Touch (2 × 8 counts)
- Figure 8 (2 × 8 counts)
- Figure 8 Bouncing (2 × 8 counts)
- 2 Foot Jump Sprint (20 seconds)
- Out of the rope
- Recover with Resting Moves (30 seconds to 1 minute)

Recovery Jump

- Figure 8 (2 × 8 counts)
- 2 Turns to Each Side (2 × 8 counts)
- 2 Turns Step Touch (2 × 8 counts)
- Figure 8 (2 × 8 counts)
- Figure 8 Bouncing (2 × 8 counts)
- 2 Foot Jump (2 × 8 counts)
- Alternating Foot (2 × 8 counts)
- Out of the rope
- Recover with Resting Moves (30 seconds to 1 minute)

Combination

- Figure 8 (2 × 8 counts)
- 2 Turns to Each Side (2 × 8 counts)
- 2 Turns Step Touch (2 × 8 counts)
- Figure 8 (2 × 8 counts)
- Figure 8 Bouncing (2 × 8 counts)
- 2 Foot Jump (2 × 8)
- Combination (1 or 2 sets)
  - 2 Foot Jump (8 counts)
  - Run (8 counts)
  - 2 Foot Jump (8 counts)
  - Alternating Foot (8 counts)
- Out of the rope

- Recover with Resting Moves (30 seconds to 1 minute)

Long Jump

- Figure 8 (2 × 8 counts)
- 2 Turns to Each Side (2 × 8 counts)
- 2 Turns Step Touch (2 × 8 counts)
- Figure 8 (2 × 8 counts)
- Figure 8 Bouncing (2 × 8 counts)
- 2 Foot Jump (5 × 8 counts)
- Alternating Foot (5 × 8 counts)
- FreeStyle Jumping (30 seconds)
- Out of the rope
- Recover with Resting Moves (30 seconds to 1 minute)

Cooldown

- FreeStyle Rope Turns (1 minute)
- Figure 8 (2 × 8 counts)
- 2 Turns to Each Side (4 × 8 counts)
- 2 Turns Step Touch (4 × 8 counts)
- Figure 8 (2 × 8 counts)
- Figure 8, right hand (8 counts)
- Figure 8, left hand (8 counts)

Strength

- Abdominals (2 to 3 sets)
  - Crunches (8 repetitions)
  Be sure to take a short break between crunch sets.

Cooldown Stretch, Standing (No Rope)

- Neck: head rolls (8 repetitions)
- Shoulders: shoulder circles, front and back (8 repetitions each direction)
- Triceps: arms cocked behind head, right and left (holding 10 counts each side)

- Chest: hands clasped behind the back (holding 10 counts)
- Side and back: waist bend, right and left (holding 10 counts each side)
- Hamstrings: standing stretch, right and left (holding 10 counts each side)
- Calves: calf stretch, right and left (holding 10 counts each side)
- Ankles and feet: ankle circles, right and left (8 repetitions each side)
- Inhale 4 counts/exhale 4 counts (2 repetitions)

Workout 3

Warm-up

- FreeStyle Rope Turns (1 minute)
- Figure 8 (4 × 8 counts)
- 2 Turns to Each Side (4 × 8 counts)
- Figure 8 (4 × 8 counts)
- Figure 8 Bouncing (4 × 8 counts)
- 2 Foot Jump (2 × 8 counts)
- Figure 8 (2 × 8 counts)
- Figure 8 Bouncing (2 × 8 counts)
- 2 Foot Jump (2 × 8 counts)
- FreeStyle Jumping (20 seconds)
- Out of the rope
- Recover with Resting Moves (20 seconds)
- Figure 8, right hand (8 counts)
- Figure 8, left hand (8 counts)

Warm-up Stretch (No Rope)

- Inhale 4 counts/exhale 4 counts (2 repetitions)
- Neck: head rotation (8 repetitions)
- Neck: head rolls (8 repetitions)

- Shoulders: shoulder circles, front and back (8 repetitions each direction)
- Triceps: arms across the body, right and left (holding 10 counts each side)
- Chest: hands clasped behind the back (holding 10 counts)
- Back: flex and extend (8 repetitions)
- Side and back: waist bend, right and left (holding 10 counts each side)
- Hamstrings: standing stretch, right and left (holding 10 counts each side)
- Groin and hips: runner's stretch, right and left (holding 10 counts each side)
- Hips and lower back: hip circles, right and left (8 repetitions each side)
- Ankles, feet, calves, and shins: roll front and back (8 repetitions)
- Calves: calf stretch, right and left (holding 10 counts each side)
- Shins: toe taps, right and left (16 repetitions each side)
- Ankles and feet: ankle circles, right and left (8 repetitions each side)

Jump 1

- FreeStyle Rope Turns (4 × 8 counts)
- Figure 8 (2 × 8 counts)
- 2 Turns to Each Side (2 × 8 counts)
- 2 Turns Step Touch (2 × 8 counts)
- Figure 8 (2 × 8 counts)
- Figure 8 Bouncing (2 × 8 counts)
- 2 Foot Jump (2 × 8 counts)
- Alternating Foot (2 × 8 counts)
- FreeStyle Jumping (20 seconds)
- Out of the rope
- Recover with Resting Moves (30 seconds to 1 minute)

Jump 2

- Figure 8 (2 × 8 counts)
- 2 Turns to Each Side (2 × 8 counts)
- 2 Turns Step Touch (2 × 8 counts)
- Figure 8 (2 × 8 counts)
- Figure 8 Bouncing (2 × 8 counts)
- 2 Foot Jump (3 × 8 counts)
- Boxer Shuffle (3 × 8 counts)
- FreeStyle Jumping (20 seconds)
- Out of the rope
- Recover with Resting Moves (30 seconds to 1 minute)

Sprint Jump

- Figure 8 (2 × 8 counts)
- 2 Turns to Each Side (2 × 8 counts)
- 2 Turns Step Touch (2 × 8 counts)
- Figure 8 (2 × 8 counts)
- Figure 8 Bouncing (2 × 8 counts)
- 2 Foot Jump Sprint (10 seconds)
- Alternating Foot Sprint (10 seconds)
- Out of the rope
- Recover with Resting Moves (30 seconds to 1 minute)

Recovery Jump

- Figure 8 (2 × 8 counts)
- 2 Turns to Each Side (2 × 8 counts)
- 2 Turns Step Touch (2 × 8 counts)
- Figure 8 (2 × 8 counts)
- Figure 8 Bouncing (2 × 8 counts)
- 2 Foot Jump (2 × 8 counts)
- Alternating Foot (2 × 8 counts)
- Out of the rope
- Recover with Resting Moves (30 seconds to 1 minute)

Combination

- Figure 8 (2 × 8 counts)
- 2 Turns to Each Side (2 × 8 counts)
- 2 Turns Step Touch (2 × 8 counts)
- Figure 8 (2 × 8 counts)
- Figure 8 Bouncing (2 × 8 counts)
- 2 Foot Jump (2 × 8 counts)
- Combination (1 or 2 sets)
  - 2 Foot Jump (8 counts)
  - Slalom (8 counts)
  - 2 Foot Jump (8 counts)
  - Run (8 counts)
- Out of the rope
- Recover with Resting Moves (30 seconds to 1 minute)

Long Jump

- Figure 8 (2 × 8 counts)
- 2 Turns to Each Side (2 × 8 counts)
- 2 Turns Step Touch (2 × 8 counts)
- Figure 8 (2 × 8 counts)
- Figure 8 Bouncing (2 × 8 counts)
- 2 Foot Jump (5 × 8 counts)
- Alternating Foot (5 × 8 counts)
- FreeStyle Jumping (30 seconds)
- Out of the rope
- Recover with Resting Moves (30 seconds to 1 minute)

Cooldown

- FreeStyle Rope Turns (1 minute)
- Figure 8 (2 × 8 counts)
- 2 Turns to Each Side (4 × 8 counts)
- 2 Turns Step Touch (4 × 8 counts)
- Figure 8 (2 × 8 counts)

- Figure 8, right hand (8 counts)
- Figure 8, left hand (8 counts)

Strength

- Arms and chest (2 to 3 sets)
  - Push-ups (8 repetitions)
  Be sure to take a short break between push-up sets.

Cooldown Stretch, Standing (No Rope)

- Neck: head rolls (8 repetitions)
- Shoulders: shoulder circles, front and back (8 repetitions each direction)
- Triceps: arms cocked behind head, right and left (holding 10 counts each side)
- Chest: hands clasped behind the back (holding 10 counts)
- Side and back: waist bend, right and left (holding 10 counts each side)
- Hamstrings: standing stretch, right and left (holding 10 counts each side)
- Calves: calf stretch, right and left (holding 10 counts each side)
- Ankles and feet: ankle circles, right and left (8 repetitions each side)
- Inhale 4 counts/exhale 4 counts (2 repetitions)

Workout 4

Warm-up

- FreeStyle Rope Turns (1 minute)
- Figure 8 (4 × 8 counts)
- 2 Turns to Each Side (4 × 8 counts)
- Figure 8 (4 × 8 counts)
- Figure 8 Bouncing (4 × 8 counts)
- 2 Foot Jump (2 × 8 counts)

- Figure 8 (2 × 8 counts)
- Figure 8 Bouncing (2 × 8 counts)
- 2 Foot Jump (2 × 8 counts)
- FreeStyle Jumping (20 seconds)
- Out of the rope
- Recover with Resting Moves (20 seconds)
- Figure 8, right hand (8 counts)
- Figure 8, left hand (8 counts)

Warm-up Stretch (No Rope)

- Inhale 4 counts/exhale 4 counts (2 repetitions)
- Neck: head rotation (8 repetitions)
- Neck: head rolls (8 repetitions)
- Shoulders: shoulder circles, front and back (8 repetitions each direction)
- Triceps: arms across the body, right and left (holding 10 counts each side)
- Chest: hands clasped behind the back (holding 10 counts)
- Back: flex and extend (8 repetitions)
- Side and back: waist bend, right and left (holding 10 counts each side)
- Hamstrings: standing stretch, right and left (holding 10 counts each side)
- Groin and hips: runner's stretch, right and left (holding 10 counts each side)
- Hips and lower back: hip circles, right and left (8 repetitions each side)
- Ankles, feet, calves, and shins: roll front and back (8 repetitions)
- Calves: calf stretch, right and left (holding 10 counts each side)
- Shins: toe taps, right and left (16 repetitions each side)
- Ankles and feet: ankle circles, right and left (8 repetitions each side)

Jump 1

- FreeStyle Rope Turns (4 × 8 counts)
- Figure 8 (2 × 8 counts)
- 2 Turns to Each Side (2 × 8 counts)
- 2 Turns Step Touch (2 × 8 counts)
- Figure 8 (2 × 8 counts)
- Figure 8 Bouncing (2 × 8 counts)
- 2 Foot Jump (2 × 8 counts)
- Run (2 × 8 counts)
- FreeStyle Jumping (20 seconds)
- Out of the rope
- Recover with Resting Moves (30 seconds to 1 minute)

Jump 2

- Figure 8 (2 × 8 counts)
- 2 Turns to Each Side (2 × 8 counts)
- 2 Turns Step Touch (2 × 8 counts)
- Figure 8 (2 × 8 counts)
- Figure 8 Bouncing (2 × 8 counts)
- 2 Foot Jump (3 × 8 counts)
- Slalom (3 × 8 counts)
- FreeStyle Jumping (20 seconds)
- Out of the rope
- Recover with Resting Moves (30 seconds to 1 minute)

Sprint Jump

- Figure 8 (2 × 8 counts)
- 2 Turns to Each Side (2 × 8 counts)
- 2 Turns Step Touch (2 × 8 counts)
- Figure 8 (2 × 8 counts)
- Figure 8 Bouncing (2 × 8 counts)
- 2 Foot Jump Sprint (10 seconds)
- Run Sprint (10 seconds)

- Out of the rope
- Recover with Resting Moves (30 seconds to 1 minute)

Recovery Jump

- Figure 8 (2 × 8 counts)
- 2 Turns to Each Side (2 × 8 counts)
- 2 Turns Step Touch (2 × 8 counts)
- Figure 8 (2 × 8 counts)
- Figure 8 Bouncing (2 × 8 counts)
- 2 Foot Jump (2 × 8 counts)
- Boxer Shuffle (2 × 8 counts)
- Out of the rope
- Recover with Resting Moves (30 seconds to 1 minute)

Combination

- Figure 8 (2 × 8 counts)
- 2 Turns to Each Side (2 × 8 counts)
- 2 Turns Step Touch (2 × 8 counts)
- Figure 8 (2 × 8 counts)
- Figure 8 Bouncing (2 × 8 counts)
- 2 Foot Jump (2 × 8 counts)
- Combination (1 or 2 sets)
  - 2 Foot Jump (8 counts)
  - Front/Back (8 counts)
  - 2 Foot Jump (8 counts)
  - Boxer Shuffle (8 counts)
- Out of the rope
- Recover with Resting Moves (30 seconds to 1 minute)

Long Jump

- Figure 8 (2 × 8 counts)
- 2 Turns to Each Side (2 × 8 counts)
- 2 Turns Step Touch (2 × 8 counts)

- Figure 8 (2 × 8 counts)
- Figure 8 Bouncing (2 × 8 counts)
- 2 Foot Jump (5 × 8 counts)
- Boxer Shuffle (5 × 8 counts)
- FreeStyle Jumping (30 seconds)
- Out of the rope
- Recover with Resting Moves (30 seconds to 1 minute)

Cooldown

- FreeStyle Rope Turns (1 minute)
- Figure 8 (2 × 8 counts)
- 2 Turns to Each Side (4 × 8 counts)
- 2 Turns Step Touch (4 × 8 counts)
- Figure 8 (2 × 8 counts)
- Figure 8, right hand (8 counts)
- Figure 8, left hand (8 counts)

Strength

- Legs (2 to 3 sets)
  - Alternating Lunges (16 repetitions)
  Be sure to take a short break between lunge sets.

Cooldown Stretch, Standing (No Rope)

- Neck: head rolls (8 repetitions)
- Shoulders: shoulder circles, front and back (8 repetitions each direction)
- Triceps: arms cocked behind head, right and left (holding 10 counts each side)
- Chest: hands clasped behind the back (holding 10 counts)
- Side and back: waist bend, right and left (holding 10 counts each side)
- Hamstrings: standing stretch, right and left (holding 10 counts each side)
- Calves: calf stretch, right and left (holding 10 counts each side)
- Ankles and feet: ankle circles, right and left (8 repetitions each side)
- Inhale 4 counts/exhale 4 counts (2 repetitions)

Basic Workout Grid

Basic Workout 1	Basic Workout 2	Basic Workout 3	Basic Workout 4
Warm-up	Warm-up	Warm-up	Warm-up
Stretch	Stretch	Stretch	Stretch
Jump 1 2 Foot Jump FreeStyle	**Jump 1** 2 Foot Jump FreeStyle	**Jump 1** 2 Foot Jump Alternating Foot Freestyle	**Jump 1** 2 Foot Jump Run Freestyle
Jump 2 Run Alternating Foot FreeStyle	**Jump 2** 2 Foot Jump Run FreeStyle	**Jump 2** 2 Foot Jump Boxer Shuffle FreeStyle	**Jump 2** 2 Foot Jump Slalom FreeStyle
Sprint Jump 2 Foot Jump	**Sprint Jump** 2 Foot Jump	**Sprint Jump** 2 Foot Jump Alternating Food	**Sprint Jump** 2 Foot Jump Run
Recovery Jump 2 Foot Jump	**Recovery Jump** 2 Foot Jump Alternating Foot	**Recovery Jump** 2 Foot Jump Alternating Foot	**Recovery Jump** 2 Foot Jump Boxer Shuffle
Combination 2 Foot Jump Alternating Foot 2 Foot Jump Alternating Foot	**Combination** 2 Foot Jump Run 2 Foot Jump Alternating Foot	**Combination** 2 Foot Jump Slalom 2 Foot Jump Boxer Shuffle	**Combination** 2 Foot Jump Front/Back 2 Foot Jump Boxer Shuffle
Long Jump 2 Foot Jump	**Long Jump** 2 Foot Jump Alternating Foot	**Long Jump** 2 Foot Jump Run	**Long Jump** 2 Foot Jump Boxer Shuffle
Cooldown	Cooldown	Cooldown	Cooldown
Strength Squats	**Strength** Crunches	**Strength** Push-ups	**Strength** Alternating Lunges
Cooldown Stretch	Cooldown Stretch	Cooldown Stretch	Cooldown Stretch

Chapter 13

Intermediate Jumps

Now that you've mastered the basics, it's time to expand your jump rope repertoire. In this section you'll learn a number of Intermediate Jumps and Moves that will continue to challenge you. Be patient and remember that the most effective way to learn any new jump is to practice it for a few minutes and move on to something else. If you allow yourself to become frustrated, it will take you longer than necessary to learn the jump. Whenever appropriate, I've also included the verbal cues for these jumps (*in italics*).

Remind yourself to focus on the basics and have fun. With *RopeSport: The Ultimate Jump Rope Workout*, you're limited only by your own imagination.

The Twist

Just as with the dance move, you're going to twist your body to one side and then to the other. Concentrate on keeping your stomach tight and you'll also work your

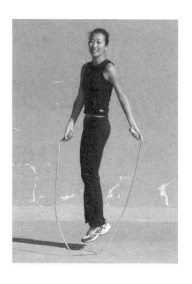

oblique muscles (the sides of your stomach) when doing the Twist.

Start in center position with the 2 Foot Jump. On the first rope rotation, twist your body to the right. On the next rotation of the rope, your body twists to the left. Continue to repeat. It's

twist / twist / twist / twist /
twist / twist / twist / twist.

A quick pointer with the Twist is to keep your hands facing straight ahead while your body is twisting from side to side. Chubby Checker, watch out!

V Jump

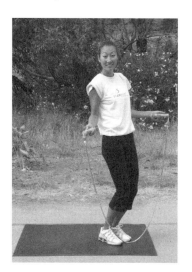

The V Jump is a great move for improving your balance and core stability. Start in center position with the 2 Foot Jump. On the first rotation of the rope, jump forward and out to the right at an angle. On the next rotation of the rope, jump back to where you started in center position. On the next rotation, jump forward and out to your left at an angle. To complete the V, jump back to where you started in center position. Continue to repeat. It's

right / center / left / center /
right / center / left / center.

High Knee Run

The High Knee Run is a modification of the regular Run. It's a very powerful jump that requires a lot of energy and simulates a training drill used by many competitive athletes to maximize speed and power development.

Start in center position with the 2 Foot Jump. Begin the Run. Whenever you're ready, bring your legs in front of you and drive your knees up as you continue to run. If you want to really push yourself, increase your speed so you're sprinting through the rope. I guarantee you'll be sucking wind in no time at all. It's

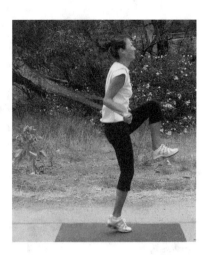

run / run / run / run / run / run / run / run.

Side to Side

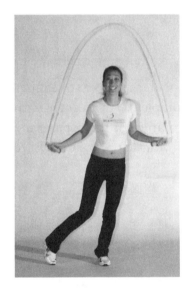

Start center with the 2 Foot Jump. On the first rotation of the rope, extend your right foot out to the side and tap your right toe. On the next rotation of the rope, bring your right foot back to center position while simultaneously extending your left foot to the side and tapping your left toe. Continue to repeat.

I like this move because it's not too difficult and you can really add your own personal flavor. It's

side / side / side / side / side / side / side / side.

Step Kick Front

I took the Step Kick straight out of aerobics class and added a rope.

The Step Kick takes four rotations of the rope to complete. Start center with a 2 Foot Jump. On the first rotation of the rope, you bounce on your left foot while your right foot comes behind and prepares to kick. On the next rotation of the rope, you kick with your right foot while

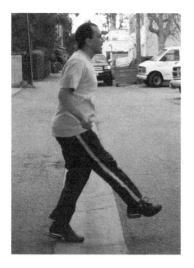

continuing to bounce on your left. On the third rotation of the rope, your right foot comes back to center and continues to bounce while your left foot comes behind you and prepares to kick. On the fourth and final rotation, kick forward with your left foot while bouncing on your right foot. Continue to repeat. It's

step / kick / step / kick / step / kick / step / kick.

The footwork for the step kick can be a little awkward at first, but just hang in there and be patient.

Step Kick Back

The Step Kick Back is very similar to the Step Kick Front. The only difference is that you kick backward instead of forward. The verbal cue is the same. It's

step / kick / step / kick / step / kick / step / kick.

Heel Back

The Heel Back is one of my personal favorites and requires four rotations of the rope to complete. Start center with the 2 Foot Jump. On the first rotation of the rope, bring your right foot behind you with your leg bent at the knee

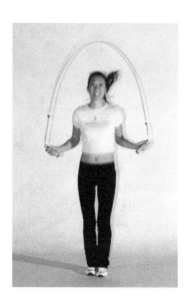
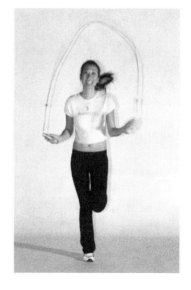

while you take one jump on your left foot. On the next rotation of the rope, bring your right foot back to the center and take one jump with both feet. On the third rotation, your left foot comes behind you with your leg bent at the knee while you take one jump on your right foot. To complete the move, bring your left foot back to center and take one jump with both feet. Continue to repeat. It's

back / center / back / center /
back / center / back / center.

Heel Together

Start in center position with the 2 Foot Jump. On the first rope rotation, extend your right foot forward and tap your right heel. On the next rope rotation, bring your right foot back to center position and take one jump with both feet. On the third rotation, extend your left foot forward and tap your left heel. Bring your left foot back to center position and take a jump with both feet on the final rotation. Continue to repeat. It's

heel / center / heel / center /
heel / center / heel / center.

Foot Cross

Start with the 2 Foot Jump. Whenever you're ready, jump into the Straddle Position (see chapter 10, "Basic Jumps").

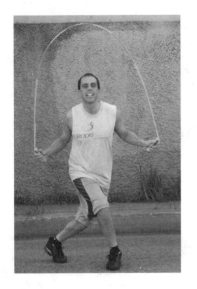 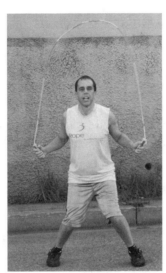

Your feet are spread apart as if you were doing a jumping jack. On the next rotation of the rope, your feet move into a crossed position with your right foot forward and your left foot behind. On the next rotation, uncross your feet into the straddle position. To complete the move, on the final rotation cross your feet again with your left foot forward and your right foot behind. Continue to repeat. It's

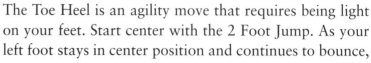

straddle / cross / straddle / cross /
straddle / cross / straddle / cross.

The Foot Cross looks cool and is a jump that will really impress your friends.

Toe Heel

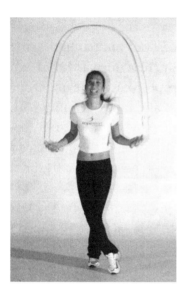
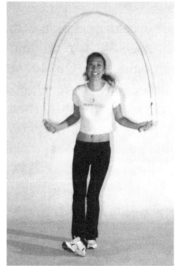

The Toe Heel is an agility move that requires being light on your feet. Start center with the 2 Foot Jump. As your left foot stays in center position and continues to bounce, you alternate by tapping your right toe on the first rotation of the rope, followed by tapping your right heel on the next rotation. Continue to repeat. It's

toe / heel / toe / heel /
toe / heel / toe / heel.

Do the same thing on the other side with your right foot continuing to bounce in center position while you alternate tapping your left heel and left toe.

Holding Cross

The Holding Cross is a fun, stylized move and a variation on the regular Cross. However, instead of uncrossing your arms each time the rope passes behind you and crossing them as it comes in front (as you do with the regular Cross), with the Holding Cross you keep your arms in the crossed position as the rope continues to rotate. It's that simple. It's

cross / cross / cross / cross /
cross / cross / cross / cross.

Double Bounce

Until now you've learned many jumps by alternating the position of your feet with every rotation of the rope. For example, when you learned the Run you ran on your right foot and then your left foot (or vice versa).

A fun and easy variation is to keep your feet in the same position as the rope rotates a second time. With the Run, for example, try taking two bounces with your right foot, followed by two bounces with your left foot. Or with the Lunge, take two bounces with your right foot forward and left foot behind, followed by two bounces with your left foot forward and your right foot behind. It's just one more way to add variety and keep things interesting.

Sprint Intervals

Sprint Intervals will optimize your cardio, burn tons of fat, and lead to significant improvements in hand and foot speed. That's why they are an integral part of training routines for world-class athletes whose careers depend on performing at the highest possible level.

With Sprint Intervals you jump as fast as you can for short periods of 20 to 60 seconds. The three jumps I normally recommend for Sprint Intervals are the 2 Foot Jump, the Run, and the Boxer Shuffle. However, you can do them with other jumps, too. By changing tempo with a sudden burst of speed and jumping fast until you can't any longer, you will increase the functional capacity of your heart and lungs. This will undoubtedly give you a competitive edge in sports such as tennis or basketball. When your opponents are slowing down, you'll be just warming up. Another benefit you'll get from training with Sprint Intervals is improvement in your hand and foot speed, something that's important in almost any sport you can think of. Finally, by pushing yourself to the limit with Sprint Intervals, you'll be burning a ton of fat and calories.

Half Figure 8 Entrance

Start with the Basic 2 Foot Jump. When the rope passes over your head, your right hand crosses over to the left side of your torso so that it's positioned on top of your left hand. However, instead of transitioning to a Figure 8 Rope Turn, bring your right hand back to where it started on your right side. By doing so, you'll be "opening" the rope by separating the handles, at which time you'll jump back into the rope and continue with a Basic 2 Foot Jump. This completes the Half Figure 8 Entrance.

A very common mistake with the Half Figure 8 Entrance is bringing the crossing hand *under* the hand that's at your side instead of over. If that happens you'll inevitably get tangled up in the rope. Also, be sure to keep the hand that's at your side stationary, and don't move it while the other hand crosses over. If the hand that is at your side moves, it will prevent you from making a clean, relaxed entrance back into the rope.

While I suggest that you start practicing the Half Figure 8 Entrance with a 2 Foot Jump, you can also do it with many other jumps, including the Alternating Foot, the Basic Run, the Boxer Shuffle, or the Lunge. After you get a feel for the Half Figure 8 Entrance, try increasing your speed and doing it at a much faster pace. You can really whip the rope by generating a lot of speed from the crossing hand, making this a very powerful move.

Backward Figure 8 Entrance

The Backward Figure 8 Entrance is done exactly like the forward entrance except in the reverse direction. Begin by doing a Backward Figure 8 Rope Turn. When the rope passes over your head, separate the handles and jump through the rope into a Backward 2 Foot Jump. Make sure you keep the handles together and don't let them separate until the rope passes over your head. If they separate too early, it will throw off your timing and cause you to miss.

Backward Variations

Now it's time to really challenge yourself and literally double the jumps you can incorporate into your workout by executing all your jumps backward. Remind yourself that jumping backward is no harder than jumping forward and that virtually every jump can and should be done backward. Practice a few minutes each workout, be patient, and before you know it you'll be jumping backward like a pro.

Doubles

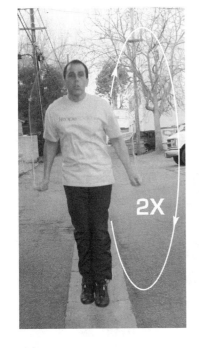

Instead of the rope rotating one time for each time your feet land, with Doubles the rope rotates twice per jump. Start with the 2 Foot Jump. Whenever you're ready, snap your wrists so the rope rotates two times before your feet hit the ground again. Now, what I want you to focus on is how fast you rotate your wrists and not how high you jump. Avoid bringing your knees up when you elevate, something that I see all too frequently when beginners are first learning Doubles. If you jump too high you'll land a lot harder than necessary and use a lot of excess energy. At first try successfully executing one Double at a time before stringing a few together consecutively. Keep in mind that doing Doubles—and almost every other jump—is about proper technique and timing. It's all in the wrist snap. It's

snap snap / snap snap / snap snap / snap snap / snap snap / snap snap / snap snap / snap snap.

Doubles are an intense, high-impact move that'll do wonders for your speed and power development, cardiovascular conditioning, explosiveness, vertical leaping ability, and so on. And because they require increased rotation speed, you should also consider giving your speed rope a try.

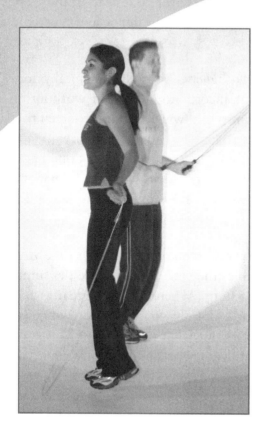

Intermediate Jump Combinations

Once you've learned the Basic Jump Combinations and are ready to progress to the next level, here are some Intermediate Jump Combinations that are a little more challenging. All jump combinations are written out in sets of eight counts. As with the Basic Jump Combinations, you can make combinations longer by either repeating each individual jump for an additional eight counts or repeating the entire combination. Continue to utilize Resting Moves to recover and catch your breath whenever necessary!

Intermediate Jump Combination 1

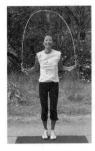 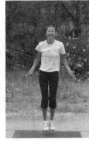

2 Foot Jump

jump / jump / jump / jump /
jump / jump / jump / jump

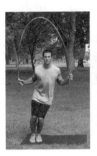 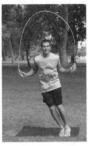

Slalom

right / left / right / left / right / left / right / left

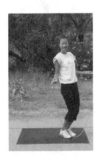

V Jump

right / center / left / center /
right / center / left / center

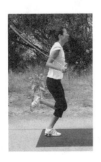

Run

run right / run left / run right / run left /
run right / run left / run right / run left

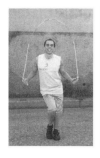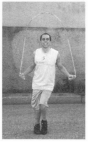

Alternating Foot

hop right / hop left / hop right / hop left /
hop right / hop left / hop right / hop left

Intermediate Jump Combination 2

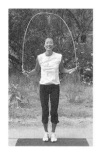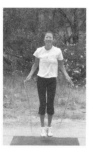

2 Foot Jump

jump / jump / jump / jump /
jump / jump / jump / jump

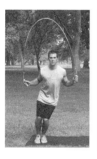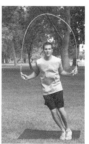

Slalom

right / left / right / left / right / left / right / left

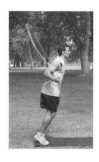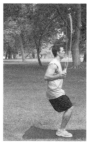

Front/Back

front / back / front / back / front / back / front / back

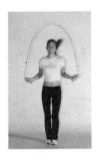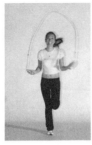

Heel Back

back right / center / back left / center /
back right / center / back left / center

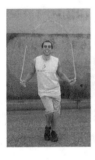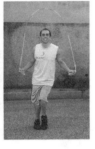

Alternating Foot

hop right / hop left / hop right / hop left /
hop right / hop left / hop right / hop left

Intermediate Jump Combination 3

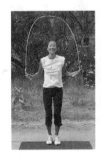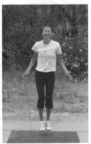

2 Foot Jump

jump / jump / jump / jump /
jump / jump / jump / jump

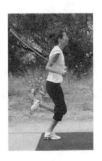

Run

run right / run left / run right / run left /
run right / run left / run right / run left

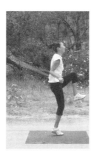

High Knee Run

run right / run left / run right / run left /
run right / run left / run right / run left

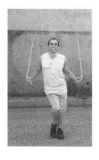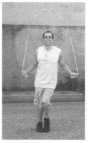

Alternating Foot

hop right / hop left / hop right / hop left /
hop right / hop left / hop right / hop left

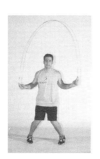

Straddle

out / center / out / center / out / center / out / center

Intermediate Jump Combination 4

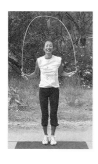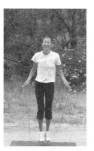

2 Foot Jump

jump / jump / jump / jump /
jump / jump / jump / jump

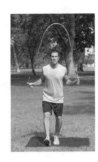

Boxer Shuffle

dig right / dig left / dig right / dig left /
dig right / dig left / dig right / dig left

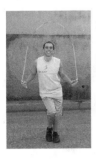 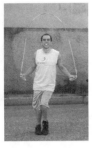

Alternating Foot

hop right / hop left / hop right / hop left /
hop right / hop left / hop right / hop left

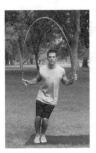 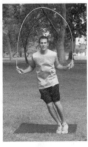

Slalom

right / left / right / left / right / left / right / left

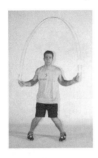

Straddle

out / center / out / center / out / center / out / center

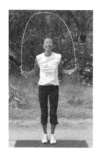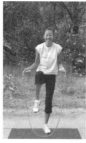

Alternating Knee Up

right knee up / center / left knee up / center /
right knee up / center / left knee up / center

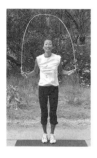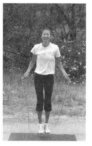

2 Foot Jump

jump / jump / jump / jump /
jump / jump / jump / jump

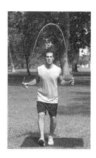

Boxer Shuffle

dig right / dig left / dig right / dig left /
dig right / dig left / dig right / dig left

Intermediate Jump Combination 5

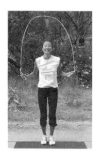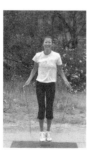

2 Foot Jump

jump / jump / jump / jump /
jump / jump / jump / jump

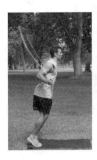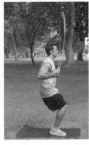

Front/Back

front / back / front / back / front / back / front / back

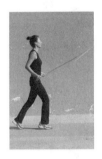

Lunge

lunge right / lunge left / lunge right / lunge left / lunge right / lunge left / lunge right / lunge left

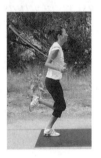

Run

run right / run left / run right / run left / run right / run left / run right / run left

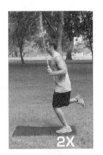

Run, Double Bounce

run right / hop right / run left / hop left / run right / hop right / run left / hop left

Intermediate Jump Combination 6

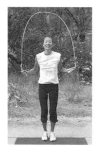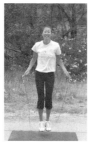

2 Foot Jump

jump / jump / jump / jump /
jump / jump / jump / jump

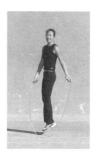

Twist

twist right / twist left / twist right / twist left /
twist right / twist left / twist right / twist left

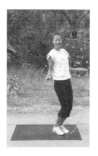

V Jump

right / center / left / center /
right / center / left / center

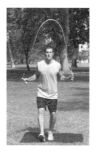

Boxer Shuffle

dig right / dig left / dig right / dig left /
dig right / dig left / dig right / dig left

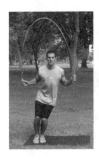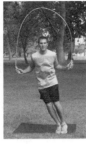

Slalom

right / left / right / left / right / left / right / left

Intermediate Jump Combination 7

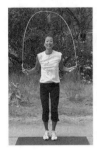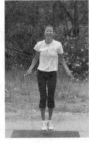

2 Foot Jump

jump / jump / jump / jump /
jump / jump / jump / jump

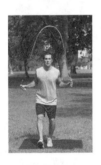

Boxer Shuffle

dig right / dig left / dig right / dig left /
dig right / dig left / dig right / dig left

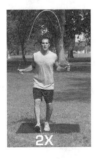

Boxer Shuffle, Double Bounce

dig right / dig right / dig left / dig left /
dig right / dig right / dig left / dig left

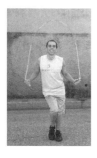 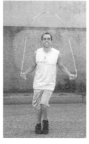

Alternating Foot

*hop right / hop left / hop right / hop left /
hop right / hop left / hop right / hop left*

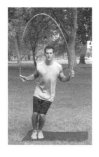 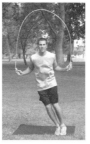

Slalom

right / left / right / left / right / left / right / left

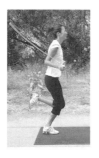

Run

*run right / run left / run right / run left /
run right / run left / run right / run left*

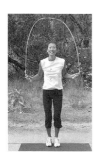 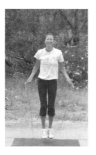

2 Foot Jump

*jump / jump / jump / jump /
jump / jump / jump / jump*

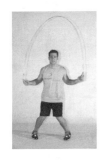

Straddle

out / center / out / center / out / center / out / center

Intermediate Jump Combination 8

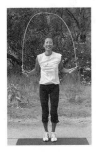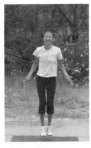

2 Foot Jump

jump / jump / jump / jump /
jump / jump / jump / jump

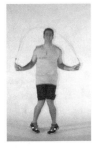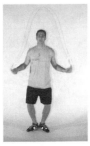

Toe In/Toe Out

in / out / in / out / in / out / in / out

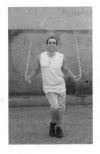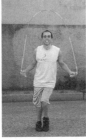

Alternating Foot

hop right / hop left / hop right / hop left /
hop right / hop left / hop right / hop left

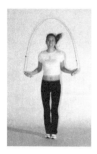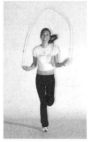

Heel Back

back right / center / back left / center /
back right / center / back left / center

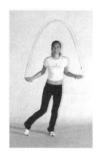

Side to Side

tap right / tap left / tap right / tap left /
tap right / tap left / tap right / tap left

Intermediate Jump Combination 9

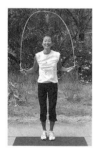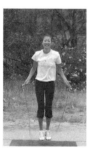

2 Foot Jump

jump / jump / jump / jump /
jump / jump / jump / jump

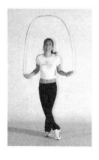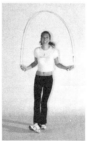

Toe Heel, right foot

right toe / right heel / right toe / right heel /
right toe / right heel / right toe / right heel

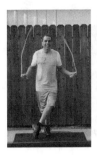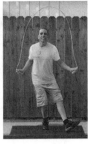

Toe Heel, left foot

left toe / left heel / left toe / left heel /
left toe / left heel / left toe / left heel

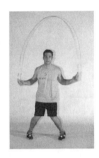

Straddle

out / center / out / center / out / center / out / center

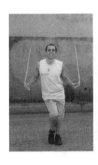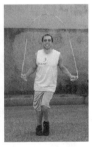

Alternating Foot

hop right / hop left / hop right / hop left /
hop right / hop left / hop right / hop left

Intermediate Jump Combination 10

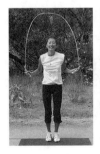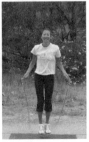

2 Foot Jump

jump / jump / jump / jump /
jump / jump / jump / jump

Intermediate Jump Combinations

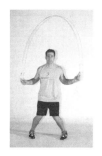

Straddle

out / center / out / center / out / center / out / center

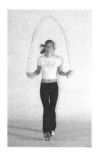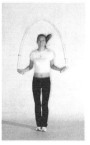

Heel Together

dig right / center / dig left / center /
dig right / center / dig left / center

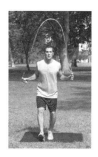

Boxer Shuffle

dig right / dig left / dig right / dig left /
dig right / dig left / dig right / dig left

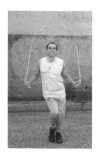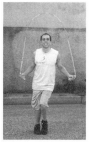

Alternating Foot

hop right / hop left / hop right / hop left /
hop right / hop left / hop right / hop left

Intermediate Jump Combination Bonus #1: Vertical Movement

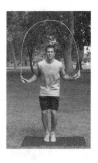

2 Foot Jump, in place

jump / jump / jump / jump /
jump / jump / jump / jump

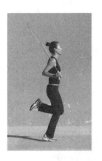

Run, traveling forward

run right / run left / run right / run left /
run right / run left / run right / run left

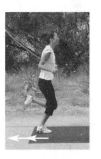

Heel Back, traveling backward

back right / center / back left / center /
back right / center / back left / center

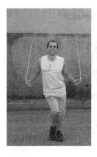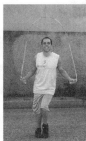

Alternating Foot, traveling forward

hop right / hop left / hop right / hop left /
hop right / hop left / hop right / hop left

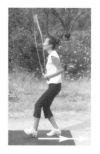

Boxer Shuffle, traveling backward

dig right / dig left / dig right / dig left /
dig right / dig left / dig right / dig left

Intermediate Jump Combination Bonus #2: Increased Difficulty

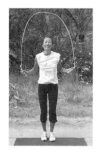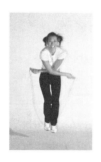

2 Foot Jump

jump / jump / jump / jump /
jump / jump / jump / jump

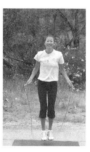

Crosses

cross / uncross / cross / uncross /
cross / uncross / cross / uncross

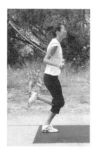

Run

run right / run left / run right / run left /
run right / run left / run right / run left

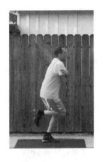

Run with Crosses

cross arms, run right / uncross arms, run left /
cross arms, run right / uncross arms, run left /
cross arms, run right / uncross arms, run left /
cross arms, run right / uncross arms, run left

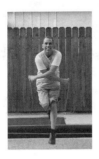

Run with Holding Crosses

cross, run right / hold cross, run left /
hold cross, run right / hold cross, run left /
hold cross, run right / hold cross, run left /
hold cross, run right / uncross, run left

Chapter 15

Intermediate RopeSport Workouts

(125–130 beats per minute; 25–40 minutes)

U se the following workouts on a weekly rotation. They should last you about a month. As your skill level improves, feel free to mix and match to fit your own unique style. Please note that the Intermediate Workout Grid on page 145 is meant to be used as a quick reference guide. The grid does not include Resting Moves between the jump sections or specific moves for the Stretches or Cooldowns. Please refer to the workout section below for a detailed list of the Stretches, Resting Moves, and Cooldowns.

Workout 1

Warm-up

- FreeStyle Rope Turns (1 minute)
- Figure 8 (4 × 8 counts)

- 2 Turns to Each Side (4 × 8 counts)
- Figure 8 (4 × 8 counts)
- Figure 8 Bouncing (4 × 8 counts)
- 2 Foot Jump (3 × 8 counts)
- FreeStyle Jumping (20 seconds)

- Out of the rope
- Recovery with Resting Moves (20 seconds)
- 2 Turns to Each Side (4 × 8 counts)
- Figure 8 (4 × 8 counts)
- Figure 8 Bouncing (4 × 8 counts)
- 2 Foot Jump (3 × 8 counts)
- FreeStyle Jumping (20 seconds)
- Out of the rope
- Recover with Resting Moves (20 seconds)
- Figure 8, right hand (8 counts)
- Figure 8, left hand (8 counts)

Warm-up Stretch (No Rope)

- Inhale 4 counts/exhale 4 counts (2 repetitions)
- Neck: head rotation (8 repetitions)
- Neck: head rolls (8 repetitions)
- Shoulders: shoulder circles, front and back (8 repetitions each direction)
- Triceps: arms across the body, right and left (holding 10 counts each side)
- Chest: hands clasped behind the back (holding 10 counts)
- Back: flex and extend (8 repetitions)
- Side and back: waist bend, right and left (holding 10 counts each side)
- Hamstrings: standing stretch, right and left (holding 10 counts each side)
- Calves: calf stretch, right and left (holding 10 counts each side)
- Groin and hips: runner's stretch, right and left (holding 10 counts each side)
- Hips and lower back: hip circles, right and left (8 repetitions each side)
- Ankles, feet, calves, and shins: roll front and back (8 repetitions)

- Shins: toe taps, right and left (16 repetitions each side)
- Ankles and feet: ankle circles, right and left (8 repetitions each side)

Jump 1

- FreeStyle Rope Turns (4 × 8 counts)
- Figure 8 (2 × 8 counts)
- 2 Turns to Each Side (2 × 8 counts)
- 2 Turns Step Touch (2 × 8 counts)
- Figure 8 (2 × 8 counts)
- Figure 8 Bouncing (2 × 8 counts)
- 2 Foot Jump (3 × 8 counts)
- Alternating Foot (3 × 8 counts)
- FreeStyle Jumping (30 seconds)
- Out of the rope
- Recover with Resting Moves (30 seconds to 1 minute)

Jump 2

- Figure 8 (2 × 8 counts)
- 2 Turns to Each Side (2 × 8 counts)
- 2 Turns Step Touch (2 × 8 counts)
- Figure 8 (2 × 8 counts)
- Figure 8 Bouncing (2 × 8 counts)
- 2 Foot Jump (4 × 8 counts)
- Run (4 × 8 counts)
- FreeStyle Jumping (30 seconds)
- Out of the rope
- Recover with Resting Moves (30 seconds to 1 minute)

Sprint Jump

- Figure 8 (2 × 8 counts)
- 2 Turns to Each Side (2 × 8 counts)

- 2 Turns Step Touch (2 × 8 counts)
- Figure 8 (2 × 8 counts)
- Figure 8 Bouncing (2 × 8 counts)
- 2 Foot Jump Sprint (30 seconds)
- Out of the rope
- Recover with Resting Moves (30 seconds to 1 minute)

Recovery Jump

- Figure 8 (2 × 8 counts)
- 2 Turns to Each Side (2 × 8 counts)
- 2 Turns Step Touch (2 × 8 counts)
- Figure 8 (2 × 8 counts)
- Figure 8 Bouncing (2 × 8 counts)
- 2 Foot Jump (6 × 8 counts)
- Out of the rope
- Recover with Resting Moves (30 seconds to 1 minute)

Combination

- Figure 8 (2 × 8 counts)
- 2 Turns to Each Side (2 × 8 counts)
- 2 Turns Step Touch (2 × 8 counts)
- Figure 8 (2 × 8 counts)
- Figure 8 Bouncing (2 × 8 counts)
- 2 Foot Jump (2 × 8 counts)
- Combination (1 to 3 sets)
  - 2 Foot Jump (8 counts)
  - Slalom (8 counts)
  - Front/Back (8 counts)
  - Lunge (8 counts)
  - Alternating Foot (8 counts)
- Out of the rope
- Recover with Resting Moves (30 seconds to 1 minute)

Jump 3

- Figure 8 (2 × 8 counts)
- 2 Turns to Each Side (2 × 8 counts)
- 2 Turns Step Touch (2 × 8 counts)
- Figure 8 (2 × 8 counts)
- Figure 8 Bouncing (2 × 8 counts)
- 2 Foot Jump (5 × 8 counts)
- Run (5 × 8 counts)
- FreeStyle Jumping (30 seconds)
- Out of the rope
- Recover with Resting Moves (30 seconds to 1 minute)

Long Jump

- Figure 8 (2 × 8 counts)
- 2 Turns to Each Side (2 × 8 counts)
- 2 Turns Step Touch (2 × 8 counts)
- Figure 8 (2 × 8 counts)
- Figure 8 Bouncing (2 × 8 counts)
- 2 Foot Jump (5 × 8 counts)
- Alternating Foot (5 × 8 counts)
- Boxer Shuffle (5 × 8 counts)
- FreeStyle Jumping (30 seconds)
- Out of the rope
- Recover with Resting Moves (30 seconds to 1 minute)

Cooldown

- FreeStyle Rope Turns (1 minute)
- Figure 8 (2 × 8 counts)
- 2 Turns to Each Side (4 × 8 counts)
- 2 Turns Step Touch (4 × 8 counts)
- Figure 8 (2 × 8 counts)
- Figure 8, right hand (8 counts)
- Figure 8, left hand (8 counts)

Strength

- Legs and butt (2 to 3 sets)
  - Squats (8 repetitions)
  - Squats at double speed (16 repetitions)
  Be sure to take a short break between squat sets.

Cooldown Stretch, Standing (No Rope)

- Neck: head rolls (8 repetitions)
- Shoulders: shoulder circles, front and back (8 repetitions each direction)
- Triceps: arms cocked behind head, right and left (holding 10 counts each side)
- Chest: hands clasped behind the back (holding 10 counts)
- Side and back: waist bend, right and left (holding 10 counts each side)
- Hips and lower back: hip circles, right and left (8 repetitions each direction)
- Hamstrings: standing stretch, right and left (holding 10 counts each side)
- Calves: calf stretch, right and left (holding 10 counts each side)
- Ankles and feet: ankle circles, right and left (8 repetitions each side)
- Inhale 4 counts/exhale 4 counts (2 repetitions)

Workout 2

Warm-up

- FreeStyle Rope Turns (1 minute)
- Figure 8 (4 × 8 counts)
- 2 Turns to Each Side (4 × 8 counts)
- Figure 8 (4 × 8 counts)
- Figure 8 Bouncing (4 × 8 counts)
- 2 Foot Jump (3 × 8 counts)
- FreeStyle Jumping (20 seconds)
- Out of the rope
- Recover with Resting Moves (20 seconds)
- 2 Turns to Each Side (4 × 8 counts)
- Figure 8 (4 × 8 counts)
- Figure 8 Bouncing (4 × 8 counts)
- 2 Foot Jump (3 × 8 counts)
- FreeStyle Jumping (20 seconds)
- Out of the rope
- Recover with Resting Moves (20 seconds)
- Figure 8, right hand (8 counts)
- Figure 8, left hand (8 counts)

Warm-up Stretch (No Rope)

- Inhale 4 counts/exhale 4 counts (2 repetitions)
- Neck: head rotation (8 repetitions)
- Neck: head rolls (8 repetitions)
- Shoulders: shoulder circles, front and back (8 repetitions each direction)
- Triceps: arms across the body, right and left (holding 10 counts each side)
- Chest: hands clasped behind the back (holding 10 counts)
- Back: flex and extend (8 repetitions)
- Side and back: waist bend, right and left (holding 10 counts each side)
- Hamstrings: standing stretch, right and left (holding 10 counts each side)
- Calves: calf stretch, right and left (holding 10 counts each side)
- Groin and hips: runner's stretch, right and left (holding 10 counts each side)
- Hips and lower back: hip circles, right and left (8 repetitions each side)
- Ankles, feet, calves, and shins: roll front and back (8 repetitions)

- Shins: toe taps, right and left (16 repetitions each side)
- Ankles and feet: ankle circles, right and left (8 repetitions each side)

Jump 1

- FreeStyle Rope Turns (4 × 8 counts)
- Figure 8 (2 × 8 counts)
- 2 Turns to Each Side (2 × 8 counts)
- 2 Turns Step Touch (2 × 8 counts)
- Figure 8 (2 × 8 counts)
- Figure 8 Bouncing (2 × 8 counts)
- 2 Foot Jump (3 × 8 counts)
- Slalom (3 × 8 counts)
- FreeStyle Jumping (30 seconds)
- Out of the rope
- Recover with Resting Moves (30 seconds to 1 minute)

Jump 2

- Figure 8 (2 × 8 counts)
- 2 Turns to Each Side (2 × 8 counts)
- 2 Turns Step Touch (2 × 8 counts)
- Figure 8 (2 × 8 counts)
- Figure 8 Bouncing (2 × 8 counts)
- 2 Foot Jump (4 × 8 counts)
- Straddle (4 × 8 counts)
- FreeStyle Jumping (30 seconds)
- Out of the rope
- Recover with Resting Moves (30 seconds to 1 minute)

Sprint Jump

- Figure 8 (2 × 8 counts)
- 2 Turns to Each Side (2 × 8 counts)
- 2 Turns Step Touch (2 × 8 counts)
- Figure 8 (2 × 8 counts)

- Figure 8 Bouncing (2 × 8 counts)
- 2 Foot Jump Sprint (15 seconds)
- Alternating Foot Sprint (15 seconds)
- Out of the rope
- Recover with Resting Moves (30 seconds to 1 minute)

Recovery Jump

- Figure 8 (2 × 8 counts)
- 2 Turns to Each Side (2 × 8 counts)
- 2 Turns Step Touch (2 × 8 counts)
- Figure 8 (2 × 8 counts)
- Figure 8 Bouncing (2 × 8 counts)
- 2 Foot Jump (2 × 8 counts)
- Alternating Foot (4 × 8 counts)
- Out of the rope
- Recover with Resting Moves (30 seconds to 1 minute)

Combination

- Figure 8 (2 × 8 counts)
- 2 Turns to Each Side (2 × 8 counts)
- 2 Turns Step Touch (2 × 8 counts)
- Figure 8 (2 × 8 counts)
- Figure 8 Bouncing (2 × 8 counts)
- 2 Foot Jump (2 × 8 counts)
- Combination (1 to 3 sets)
  - 2 Foot Jump (8 counts)
  - Straddle (8 counts)
  - Lunge (8 counts)
  - Basic Run (8 counts)
  - Alternating Foot (8 counts)
- Out of the rope
- Recover with Resting Moves (30 seconds to 1 minute)

Jump 3

- Figure 8 (2 × 8 counts)
- 2 Turns to Each Side (2 × 8 counts)
- 2 Turns Step Touch (2 × 8 counts)
- Figure 8 (2 × 8 counts)
- Figure 8 Bouncing (2 × 8 counts)
- 2 Foot Jump (5 × 8 counts)
- Twist (5 × 8 counts)
- FreeStyle Jumping (30 seconds)
- Out of the rope
- Recover with Resting Moves (30 seconds to 1 minute)

Long Jump

- Figure 8 (2 × 8 counts)
- 2 Turns to Each Side (2 × 8 counts)
- 2 Turns Step Touch (2 × 8 counts)
- Figure 8 (2 × 8 counts)
- Figure 8 Bouncing (2 × 8 counts)
- 2 Foot Jump (5 × 8 counts)
- Front/Back (5 × 8 counts)
- Straddle (5 × 8) counts
- FreeStyle Jumping (30 seconds)
- Out of the rope
- Recover with Resting Moves (30 seconds to 1 minute)

Cooldown

- FreeStyle Rope Turns (1 minute)
- Figure 8 (2 × 8 counts)
- 2 Turns to Each Side (4 × 8 counts)
- 2 Turns Step Touch (4 × 8 counts)
- Figure 8 (2 × 8 counts)
- Figure 8, right hand (8 counts)
- Figure 8, left hand (8 counts)

Strength

- Abdominals (2 to 3 sets)
  - Crunches (8 repetitions)
  - Rotation crunches (16 repetitions)
  Be sure to take a short break between crunch sets.

Cooldown Stretch, Standing (No Rope)

- Neck: head rolls (8 repetitions)
- Shoulders: shoulder circles, front and back (8 repetitions each direction)
- Triceps: arms cocked behind head, right and left (holding 10 counts each side)
- Chest: hands clasped behind the back (holding 10 counts)
- Side and back: waist bend, right and left (holding 10 counts each side)
- Hips and lower back: hip circles, right and left (8 repetitions each direction)
- Hamstrings: standing stretch, right and left (holding 10 counts each side)
- Calves: calf stretch, right and left (holding 10 counts each side)
- Ankles and feet: ankle circles, right and left (8 repetitions each side)
- Inhale 4 counts/exhale 4 counts (2 repetitions)

Workout 3

Warm-up

- FreeStyle Rope Turns (1 minute)
- Figure 8 (4 × 8 counts)
- 2 Turns to Each Side (4 × 8 counts)
- Figure 8 (4 × 8 counts)
- Figure 8 Bouncing (4 × 8 counts)
- 2 Foot Jump (3 × 8 counts)

- FreeStyle Jumping (20 seconds)
- Out of the rope
- Recover with Resting Moves (20 seconds)
- 2 Turns to Each Side (4 × 8 counts)
- Figure 8 (4 × 8 counts)
- Figure 8 Bouncing (4 × 8 counts)
- 2 Foot Jump (3 × 8 counts)
- FreeStyle Jumping (20 seconds)
- Out of the rope
- Recover with Resting Moves (20 seconds)
- Figure 8, right hand (8 counts)
- Figure 8, left hand (8 counts)

Warm-up Stretch (No Rope)

- Inhale 4 counts/exhale 4 counts (2 repetitions)
- Neck: head rotation (8 repetitions)
- Neck: head rolls (8 repetitions)
- Shoulders: shoulder circles, front and back (8 repetitions each direction)
- Triceps: arms across the body, right and left (holding 10 counts each side)
- Chest: hands clasped behind the back (holding 10 counts)
- Back: flex and extend (8 repetitions)
- Side and back: waist bend, right and left (holding 10 counts each side)
- Hamstrings: standing stretch, right and left (holding 10 counts each side)
- Calves: calf stretch, right and left (holding 10 counts each side)
- Groin and hips: runner's stretch, right and left (holding 10 counts each side)
- Hips and lower back: hip circles, right and left (8 repetitions each side)
- Ankles, feet, calves, and shins: roll front and back (8 repetitions)

- Shins: toe taps, right and left (16 repetitions each side)
- Ankles and feet: ankle circles, right and left (8 repetitions each side)

Jump 1

- FreeStyle Rope Turns (4 × 8 counts)
- Figure 8 (2 × 8 counts)
- 2 Turns to Each Side (2 × 8 counts)
- 2 Turns Step Touch (2 × 8 counts)
- Figure 8 (2 × 8 counts)
- Figure 8 Bouncing (2 × 8 counts)
- 2 Foot Jump (3 × 8 counts)
- Twist (3 × 8 counts)
- FreeStyle Jumping (30 seconds)
- Out of the rope
- Recover with Resting Moves (30 seconds to 1 minute)

Jump 2

- Figure 8 (2 × 8 counts)
- 2 Turns to Each Side (2 × 8 counts)
- 2 Turns Step Touch (2 × 8 counts)
- Figure 8 (2 × 8 counts)
- Figure 8 Bouncing (2 × 8 counts)
- 2 Foot Jump (4 × 8 counts)
- Lunge (4 × 8 counts)
- FreeStyle Jumping (30 seconds)
- Out of the rope
- Recover with Resting Moves (30 seconds to 1 minute)

Sprint Jump

- Figure 8 (2 × 8 counts)
- 2 Turns to Each Side (2 × 8 counts)
- 2 Turns Step Touch (2 × 8 counts)

- Figure 8 (2 × 8 counts)
- Figure 8 Bouncing (2 × 8 counts)
- 2 Foot Jump Sprint (15 seconds)
- Run Sprint (15 seconds)
- Out of the rope
- Recover with Resting Moves (30 seconds to 1 minute)

Recovery Jump

- Figure 8 (2 × 8 counts)
- 2 Turns to Each Side (2 × 8 counts)
- 2 Turns Step Touch (2 × 8 counts)
- Figure 8 (2 × 8 counts)
- Figure 8 Bouncing (2 × 8 counts)
- 2 Foot Jump (2 × 8 counts)
- Boxer Shuffle (4 × 8 counts)
- Out of the rope
- Recover with Resting Moves (30 seconds to 1 minute)

Combination

- Figure 8 (2 × 8 counts)
- 2 Turns to Each Side (2 × 8 counts)
- 2 Turns Step Touch (2 × 8 counts)
- Figure 8 (2 × 8 counts)
- Figure 8 Bouncing (2 × 8 counts)
- 2 Foot Jump (2 × 8 counts)
- Combination (1 to 3 sets)
  - 2 Foot Jump (8 counts)
  - Run (8 counts)
  - Run, Double Bounce (8 counts)
  - Straddle (8 counts)
  - Alternating Foot (8 counts)
- Out of the rope
- Recover with Resting Moves (30 seconds to 1 minute)

Jump 3

- Figure 8 (2 × 8 counts)
- 2 Turns to Each Side (2 × 8 counts)
- 2 Turns Step Touch (2 × 8 counts)
- Figure 8 (2 × 8 counts)
- Figure 8 Bouncing (2 × 8 counts)
- 2 Foot Jump (5 × 8 counts)
- V Jump (5 × 8 counts)
- FreeStyle Jumping (30 seconds)
- Out of the rope
- Recover with Resting Moves (30 seconds to 1 minute)

Long Jump

- Figure 8 (2 × 8 counts)
- 2 Turns to Each Side (2 × 8 counts)
- 2 Turns Step Touch (2 × 8 counts)
- Figure 8 (2 × 8 counts)
- Figure 8 Bouncing (2 × 8 counts)
- 2 Foot Jump (5 × 8 counts)
- Lunge (5 × 8 counts)
- Run (5 × 8 counts)
- FreeStyle Jumping (30 seconds)
- Out of the rope
- Recover with Resting Moves (30 seconds to 1 minute)

Cooldown

- FreeStyle Rope Turns (1 minute)
- Figure 8 (2 × 8 counts)
- 2 Turns to Each Side (4 × 8 counts)
- 2 Turns Step Touch (4 × 8 counts)
- Figure 8 (2 × 8 counts)
- Figure 8, right hand (8 counts)
- Figure 8, left hand (8 counts)

Strength

- Arms and chest (2 to 3 sets)
  - Slow-tempo push-ups (4 repetitions)
  - Regular-tempo push-ups (8 repetitions)

  Be sure to take a short break between push-up sets.

Cooldown Stretch, Standing (No Rope)

- Neck: head rolls (8 repetitions)
- Shoulders: shoulder circles, front and back (8 repetitions each direction)
- Triceps: arms cocked behind head, right and left (holding 10 counts each side)
- Chest: hands clasped behind the back (holding 10 counts)
- Side and back: waist bend, right and left (holding 10 counts each side)
- Hips and lower back: hip circles, right and left (8 repetitions each direction)
- Hamstrings: standing stretch, right and left (holding 10 counts each side)
- Calves: calf stretch, right and left (holding 10 counts each side)
- Ankles and feet: ankle circles, right and left (8 repetitions each side)
- Inhale 4 counts/exhale 4 counts (2 repetitions)

Workout 4

Warm-up

- FreeStyle Rope Turns (1 minute)
- Figure 8 (4 × 8 counts)
- 2 Turns to Each Side (4 × 8 counts)
- Figure 8 (4 × 8 counts)
- Figure 8 Bouncing (4 × 8 counts)
- 2 Foot Jump (3 × 8 counts)

- FreeStyle Jumping (20 seconds)
- Out of the rope
- Recover with Resting Moves (20 seconds)
- 2 Turns to Each Side (4 × 8 counts)
- Figure 8 (4 × 8 counts)
- Figure 8 Bouncing (4 × 8 counts)
- 2 Foot Jump (3 × 8 counts)
- FreeStyle Jumping (20 seconds)
- Out of the rope
- Recover with Resting Moves (20 seconds)
- Figure 8, right hand (8 counts)
- Figure 8, left hand (8 counts)

Warm-up Stretch (No Rope)

- Inhale 4 counts/exhale 4 counts (2 repetitions)
- Neck: head rotation (8 repetitions)
- Neck: head rolls (8 repetitions)
- Shoulders: shoulder circles, front and back (8 repetitions each direction)
- Triceps: arms across the body, right and left (holding 10 counts each side)
- Chest: hands clasped behind the back (holding 10 counts)
- Back: flex and extend (8 repetitions)
- Side and back: waist bend, right and left (holding 10 counts each side)
- Hamstrings: standing stretch, right and left (holding 10 counts each side)
- Calves: calf stretch, right and left (holding 10 counts each side)
- Groin and hips: runner's stretch, right and left (holding 10 counts each side)
- Hips and lower back: hip circles, right and left (8 repetitions each side)
- Ankles, feet, calves, and shins: roll front and back (8 repetitions)

- Shins: toe taps, right and left (16 repetitions each side)
- Ankles and feet: ankle circles, right and left (8 repetitions each side)

Jump 1

- FreeStyle Rope Turns (4 × 8 counts)
- Figure 8 (2 × 8 counts)
- 2 Turns to Each Side (2 × 8 counts)
- 2 Turns Step Touch (2 × 8 counts)
- Figure 8 (2 × 8 counts)
- Figure 8 Bouncing (2 × 8 counts)
- 2 Foot Jump (3 × 8 counts)
- V Jump (3 × 8 counts)
- FreeStyle Jumping (30 seconds)
- Out of the rope
- Recover with Resting Moves (30 seconds to 1 minute)

Jump 2

- Figure 8 (2 × 8 counts)
- 2 Turns to Each Side (2 × 8 counts)
- 2 Turns Step Touch (2 × 8 counts)
- Figure 8 (2 × 8 counts)
- Figure 8 Bouncing (2 × 8 counts)
- 2 Foot Jump (4 × 8 counts)
- Front/Back (4 × 8 counts)
- FreeStyle Jumping (30 seconds)
- Out of the rope
- Recover with/Resting Moves (30 seconds to 1 minute)

Sprint Jump

- Figure 8 (2 × 8 counts)
- 2 Turns to Each Side (2 × 8 counts)
- 2 Turns Step Touch (2 × 8 counts)

- Figure 8 (2 × 8 counts)
- Figure 8 Bouncing (2 × 8 counts)
- 2 Foot Jump Sprint (15 seconds)
- Boxer Shuffle Sprint (15 seconds)
- Out of the rope
- Recover with Resting Moves (30 seconds to 1 minute)

Recovery Jump

- Figure 8 (2 × 8 counts)
- 2 Turns to Each Side (2 × 8 counts)
- 2 Turns Step Touch (2 × 8 counts)
- Figure 8 (2 × 8 counts)
- Figure 8 Bouncing (2 × 8 counts)
- 2 Foot Jump (2 × 8 counts)
- Run (4 × 8 counts)
- Out of the rope
- Recover with Resting Moves (30 seconds to 1 minute)

Combination

- Figure 8 (2 × 8 counts)
- 2 Turns to Each Side (2 × 8 counts)
- 2 Turns Step Touch (2 × 8 counts)
- Figure 8 (2 × 8 counts)
- Figure 8 Bouncing (2 × 8 counts)
- 2 Foot Jump (2 × 8 counts)
- Combination (1 to 3 sets)
  - 2 Foot Jump (8 counts)
  - Slalom (8 counts)
  - Front/Back (8 counts)
  - Alternating Knee Up (8 counts)
  - Alternating Foot (8 counts)
- Out of the rope
- Recover with Resting Moves (30 seconds to 1 minute)

Jump 3

- Figure 8 (2 × 8 counts)
- 2 Turns to Each Side (2 × 8 counts)
- 2 Turns Step Touch (2 × 8 counts)
- Figure 8 (2 × 8 counts)
- Figure 8 Bouncing (2 × 8 counts)
- 2 Foot Jump (5 × 8 counts)
- Heel Back (5 × 8 counts)
- FreeStyle Jumping (30 seconds)
- Out of the rope
- Recover with Resting Moves (30 seconds to 1 minute)

Long Jump

- Figure 8 (2 × 8 counts)
- 2 Turns to Each Side (2 × 8 counts)
- 2 Turns Step Touch (2 × 8 counts)
- Figure 8 (2 × 8 counts)
- Figure 8 Bouncing (2 × 8 counts)
- 2 Foot Jump (5 × 8 counts)
- Alternating Knee Up (5 × 8 counts)
- Alternating Foot (5 × 8) counts
- FreeStyle Jumping (30 seconds)
- Out of the rope
- Recover with Resting Moves (30 seconds to 1 minute)

Cooldown

- FreeStyle Rope Turns (1 minute)
- Figure 8 (2 × 8 counts)
- 2 Turns to Each Side (4 × 8 counts)

- 2 Turns Step Touch (4 × 8 counts)
- Figure 8 (2 × 8 counts)
- Figure 8, right hand (8 counts)
- Figure 8, left hand (8 counts)

Strength

- Legs (2 to 3 sets)
  - Alternating lunges (16 repetitions)
  - Same-leg lunges, right and left (8 repetitions each side)

Be sure to take a short break between lunge sets.

Cooldown Stretch, Standing (No Rope)

- Neck: head rolls (8 repetitions)
- Shoulders: shoulder circles, front and back (8 repetitions each direction)
- Triceps: arms cocked behind head, right and left (holding 10 counts each side)
- Chest: hands clasped behind the back (holding 10 counts)
- Side and back: waist bend, right and left (holding 10 counts each side)
- Hips and lower back: hip circles, right and left (8 repetitions each direction)
- Hamstrings: standing stretch, right and left (holding 10 counts each side)
- Calves: calf stretch, right and left (holding 10 counts each side)
- Ankles and feet: ankle circles, right and left (8 repetitions each side)
- Inhale 4 counts/exhale 4 counts (2 repetitions)

Intermediate Workout Grid

Intermediate Workout 1	Intermediate Workout 2	Intermediate Workout 3	Intermediate Workout 4
Warm-up	**Warm-up**	**Warm-up**	**Warm-up**
Warm-up Stretch	**Warm-up Stretch**	**Warm-up Stretch**	**Warm-up Stretch**
Jump 1 2 Foot Jump Alternating Foot FreeStyle	**Jump 1** 2 Foot Jump Slalom FreeStyle	**Jump 1** 2 Foot Jump Twist FreeStyle	**Jump 1** 2 Foot Jump V Jump FreeStyle
Jump 2 2 Foot Jump Run FreeStyle	**Jump 2** 2 Foot Jump Straddle FreeStyle	**Jump 2** 2 Foot Jump Lunge FreeStyle	**Jump 2** 2 Foot Jump Front/Back FreeStyle
Sprint Jump 2 Foot Jump	**Sprint Jump** 2 Foot Jump Alternating Foot	**Sprint Jump** 2 Foot Jump Run	**Sprint Jump** Alternating Foot Boxer Shuffle
Recovery Jump 2 Foot Jump	**Recovery Jump** 2 Foot Jump Alternating Foot	**Recovery Jump** 2 Foot Jump Boxer Shuffle	**Recovery Jump** 2 Foot Jump Run
Combination 2 Foot Jump Slalom Front/Back Lunge Alternating Foot	**Combination** 2 Foot Jump Straddle Lunge Run Alternating Foot	**Combination** 2 Foot Jump Run Run, Double Bounce Straddle Alternating Foot	**Combination** 2 Foot Jump Slalom Front/Back Alternating Knee Up Alternating Foot
Jump 3 2 Foot Jump Run FreeStyle	**Jump 3** 2 Foot Jump Twist FreeStyle	**Jump 3** 2 Foot Jump V Jump FreeStyle	**Jump 3** 2 Foot Jump Heel Back FreeStyle
Long Jump 2 Foot Jump Alternating Foot Boxer Shuffle	**Long Jump** 2 Foot Jump Front/Back Straddle	**Long Jump** 2 Foot Jump Lunge Run	**Long Jump** 2 Foot Jump Alternating Knee Up Alternating Foot
Cooldown	**Cooldown**	**Cooldown**	**Cooldown**
Strength Squats Single/Double Time	**Strength** Crunches Basic & Rotation	**Strength** Push-ups Single/Double Time	**Strength** Alternating & Same Side Lunges
Cooldown Stretch	**Cooldown Stretch**	**Cooldown Stretch**	**Cooldown Stretch**

Chapter 16

Advanced Jumps

Now that you've progressed to the point that you're a more skilled jumper than you ever thought possible (that's right, I'm talking to *you*!), it's time to take it to the next level with some more advanced jumps and tricks. By challenging yourself even further, your metabolism will be in high gear. As a result, you'll continue to burn a huge number of calories. You'll also be maximizing a host of athletic skills, including agility, foot speed, coordination, cardiovascular endurance, and speed and power development. At the same time, you'll be able to create more combinations by incorporating an even greater number of jumps into your routines. You'll be FreeStyling like a pro. And most importantly, you'll be having a ton of fun while you get in the best shape of your life.

If you're having difficulty mastering any of these Advanced Jumps, I would highly recommend practicing without the rope to get a feel for the footwork and timing. Then add the rope when you feel comfortable doing so. In other words, this is a perfect time to utilize the Three-Step Breakdown.

Alternating High Kicks

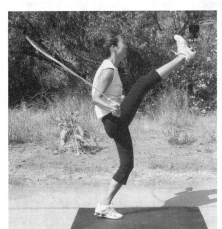

Start center with the 2 Foot Jump. Whenever you're ready, kick your right leg as high as you comfortably can in front of you and continue to bounce with your left foot in center position for one rotation of the rope. On the second rotation of the rope, your right foot comes back down and to the center. On the third rotation, kick your left leg as high as you comfortably can and continue to bounce on your right foot. On the final rotation, your left foot comes back to center position. Continue to repeat. It's

center / kick right / center / kick left /
center / kick right / center / kick left.

Can Can

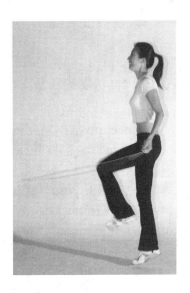 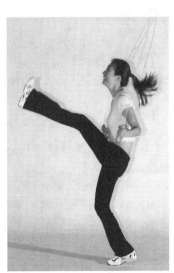

The Can Can might remind you of the step that made the Rockette dancers famous. It combines Alternating Knee Ups and Alternating High Kicks into one move.

Your left foot continues to bounce in center position as you execute a series of movements with your right leg. Start by bringing your right knee up on the first rope rotation. On the next rope rotation, your right foot comes back to center position. On the third rotation of the rope, execute a high kick with your right leg. On the fourth rotation of the rope, your right foot comes back to center position.

Repeat the same sequence of moves with your left leg as your right foot continues to bounce in center position. Continue to repeat. It's

right knee up / center / kick right / center /
left knee up / center / kick left / center.

Heel Click

Start center with the 2 Foot Jump. Whenever you're ready, jump into the Straddle position with your feet spread apart and out to the side, just like they'd be if you were doing a

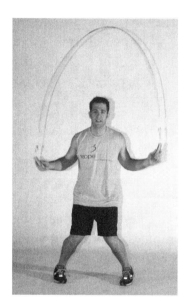 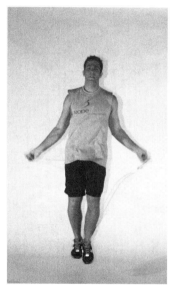

jumping jack. For every rotation of the rope, quickly bring your feet together so your heels actually touch each other, then quickly move back into Straddle position. Basically, for every rotation of the rope your feet are moving double time. Continue to repeat.

The Heel Click is a great jump for developing foot speed, something that will improve performance in many sports, including basketball, football, skiing, and tennis. It's

straddle, click /
straddle, click / straddle, click / straddle, click / straddle,
click / straddle, click / straddle, click / straddle, click.

Running Man

Do you remember the running man dance move from the 1980s? Well, here it is with a rope. It's time to get a little funky.

Start with the 2 Foot Jump. As you bring your right knee up, continue bouncing with your left foot in center position for one rotation of the rope. On the next rotation of the rope, your left foot slides behind you into a lunge as your right foot comes back to center position. On the

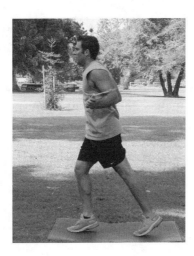
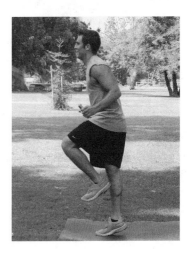

next rotation of the rope, as your right foot does one bounce in center position, bring your left knee forward and up from its position behind you. On the final rotation of the rope, your left knee comes back to center position as your right foot slides behind you. Continue to repeat. It's

lunge right / right knee up / lunge left / left knee up / lunge right / right knee up / lunge left / left knee up.

Touch Front and Back

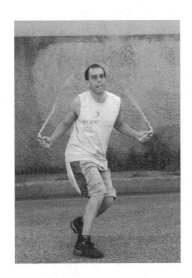
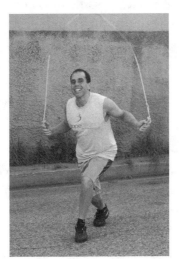

The Touch Front and Back is one of my favorite Advanced Jumps. It might take a little while to learn, but it's a cool-looking jump that you can add your own flavor to. It's also quite gentle on the body.

Start center with the 2 Foot Jump. As your left foot continues to bounce in center position, pick your right foot up and keep it in the air for one rotation of the rope. On the second rotation of the rope, bring your right shoulder forward as you turn your body to the left and touch your right foot in front of you. On the next rope rotation, raise your right foot back up and keep it in the air as you rotate your body toward the back and continue to bounce on your left foot. On the next rotation, your right foot touches behind you. Continue to repeat.

I find it helpful if you think of pivoting with your body as you execute the Touch Front and Back. And because it's a little tricky, I highly recommend trying it without the rope first in order to get a feel for the footwork and timing before you add the rope. It's

hop / touch front / hop / touch back /
hop / touch front / hop / touch back.

Knee Up Cross Over

Start center with the 2 Foot Jump. On the first rotation of the rope, bring your right knee up in front of you as your left foot continues to bounce in center position. On the second rotation of the rope, cross your right leg over so when you bring your right foot down it's tapping on the left side of your body. On the third rope rotation, bring your right knee back up and over so it's positioned squarely in front of you (where it was on the first rotation). On the final rotation of the rope your right foot moves back to center position.

Repeat the same move on the other side, with your right foot continuing to bounce in center position as your left leg does all the work. It's

knee up / cross / knee up / center /
knee up / cross / knee up / center.

Triples

A Triple is done by rotating the rope three times for each time your feet hit the ground. Triples are a *very* Advanced Jump that will really test your speed and power. And because they require maximum rotation speed, it's the perfect time to bust out your speed rope.

Start center with the 2 Foot Jump. Whenever you're ready, elevate as high as you safely can while simultaneously snapping your wrists as fast as you possibly can. As with Doubles, remember to really focus on your wrist snap. *Do not* bring your knees up in an effort to jump higher, something that can result in a lot of excess impact upon landing. Proper form and safety should always come first, no matter what jump you're doing. In fact, keeping it safe and controlled will increase the likelihood that you'll successfully execute the jump. It's

snap snap snap / snap snap snap / snap snap snap /
snap snap snap / snap snap snap / snap snap snap /
snap snap snap / snap snap snap.

Cross Variations

You can add a Cross to almost any jump. By doing so you'll increase the difficulty level, continue to challenge yourself, and add variety to your workout. For example, you can add a Cross to the Run, the Alternating Foot, Doubles, or even Triples (good luck!). Remember that while your hands are in the crossed position they should be hugging your hips and extended far past your torso, giving you a nice arc and more space to get through the rope.

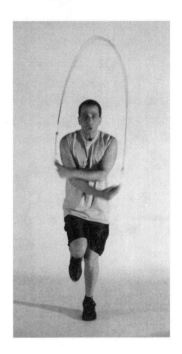

Vertical Movement

Another way to vary your workout is by moving vertically, or what we call traveling, while continuing to execute a variety of jumps. For example, try running forward and then backward. And if you want to make it even tougher, try moving forward or backward while rotating the rope either forward or backward.

Adding vertical movement while you're jumping will help to orchestrate and maximize a variety of athletic skills, including coordination, agility, timing, and foot-work. It closely mirrors the type of movements that are required in a variety of sports where you're continuously moving up and back while simultaneously catching, kicking, throwing, or striking.

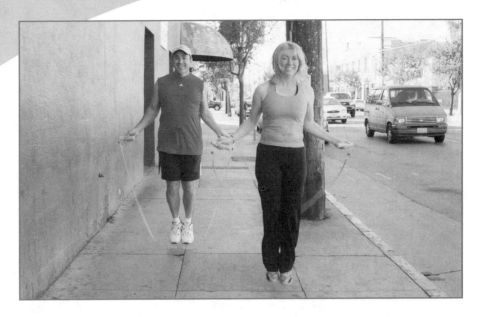

Chapter 17

Advanced Jump Combinations

Now that you're a serious roper, you're no doubt ready for the Advanced Jump Combinations! Combining six jumps or more at a time is no easy feat, clearly putting your jumping skills to the test. It's also pushing your stamina to the limit. "Got game!?"

All jump combinations are written out in sets of eight counts. Try to make it through at least two sets of combinations at a time, whether you group two different combinations together or repeat the same combination! Add Rope Turns to the combinations to really increase your upper-body workout and dazzle your friends!

Jump combinations are written out starting with the right foot, but all combinations can be done starting with either foot.

Advanced Jump Combination 1

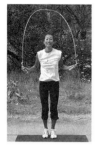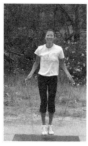

2 Foot Jump

jump / jump / jump / jump /
jump / jump / jump / jump

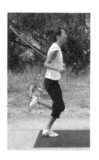

Run

run right / run left / run right / run left /
run right / run left / run right / run left

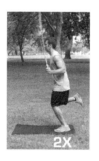

Run, Double Bounce

run right / hop right / run left / hop left /
run right / hop right / run left / hop left

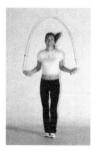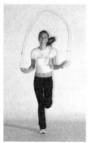

Heel Back

back right / center / back left / center /
back right / center / back left / center

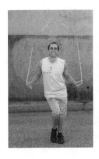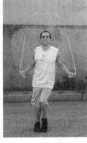

Alternating Foot

hop right / hop left / hop right / hop left /
hop right / hop left / hop right / hop left

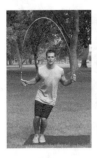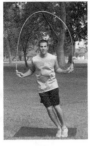

Slalom

right / left / right / left / right / left / right / left

Advanced Jump Combination 2

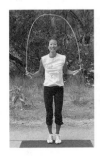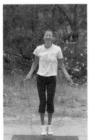

2 Foot Jump

jump / jump / jump / jump /
jump / jump / jump / jump

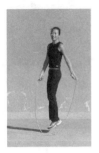

Twist

twist right / twist left / twist right / twist left /
twist right / twist left / twist right / twist left

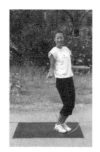

V Jump

right / center / left / center /
right / center / left / center

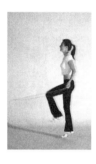 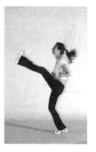

Can Can

right knee up / center / kick right / center /
left knee up / center / kick left / center

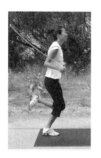

Run

run right / run left / run right / run left /
run right / run left / run right / run left

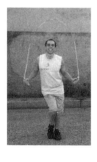 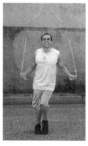

Alternating Foot

hop right / hop left / hop right / hop left /
hop right / hop left / hop right / hop left

Advanced Jump Combination 3

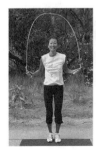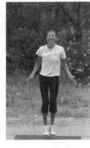

2 Foot Jump

jump / jump / jump / jump /
jump / jump / jump / jump

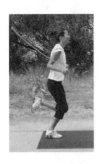

Run

run right / run left / run right / run left /
run right / run left / run right / run left

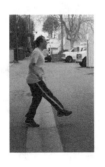

Step Kick Front

step left / kick right / step right / kick left /
step left / kick right / step right / kick left

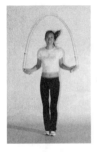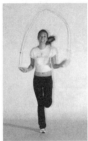

Heel Back

back right / center / back left / center /
back right / center / back left / center

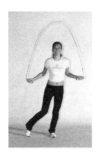

Side to Side

tap right / tap left / tap right / tap left /
tap right / tap left / tap right / tap left

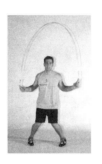

Straddle

out / center / out / center / out / center / out / center

Advanced Jump Combination 4

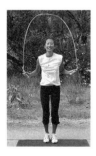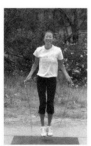

2 Foot Jump

jump / jump / jump / jump /
jump / jump / jump / jump

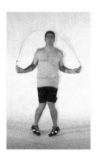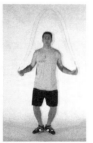

Toe In/Toe Out

in / out / in / out / in / out / in / out

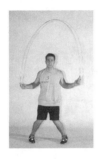

Straddle

out / center / out / center / out / center / out / center

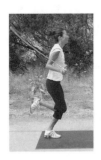

Run

run right / run left / run right / run left /
run right / run left / run right / run left

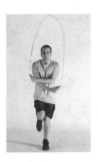

Run with Arm Crosses

cross arms, run right / uncross arms, run left /
cross arms, run right / uncross arms, run left /
cross arms, run right / uncross arms, run left /
cross arms, run right / uncross arms, run left

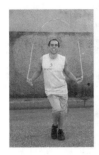 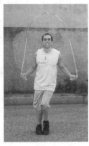

Alternating Foot

hop right / hop left / hop right / hop left /
hop right / hop left / hop right / hop left

Advanced Jump Combination 5

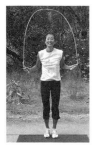 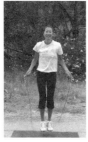

2 Foot Jump

jump / jump / jump / jump /
jump / jump / jump / jump

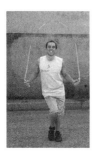 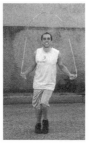

Alternating Foot

hop right / hop left / hop right / hop left /
hop right / hop left / hop right / hop left

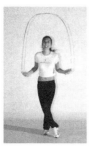 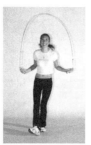

Toe Heel, right foot

right toe / right heel / right toe / right heel /
right toe / right heel / right toe / right heel

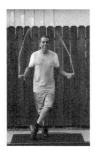 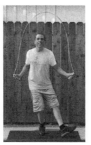

Toe Heel, left foot

left toe / left heel / left toe / left heel /
left toe / left heel / left toe / left heel

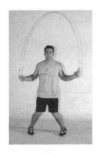

Straddle

out / center / out / center / out / center / out / center

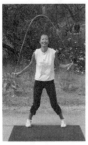
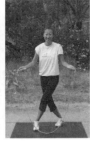

Foot Cross

straddle / cross / straddle / cross /
straddle / cross / straddle / cross

Advanced Jump Combination 6

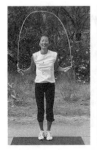
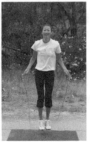

2 Foot Jump

jump / jump / jump / jump /
jump / jump / jump / jump

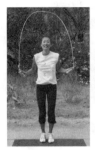
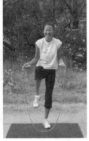

Alternating Knee Up

right knee up / center / left knee up / center /
right knee up / center / left knee up / center

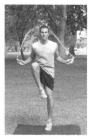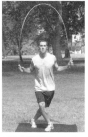

Knee Up Cross Over

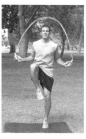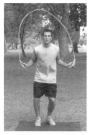

right knee up / cross touch right /
right knee up / center / left knee up /
cross touch left / left knee up / center

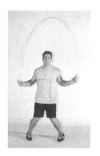

Straddle

out / center / out / center / out / center / out / center

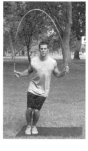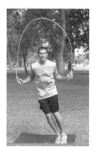

Slalom

right / left / right / left / right / left / right / left

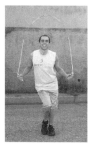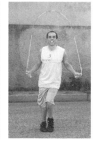

Alternating Foot

hop right / hop left / hop right / hop left /
hop right / hop left / hop right / hop left

Advanced Jump Combination 7

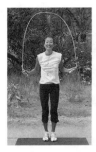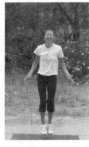

2 Foot Jump

jump / jump / jump / jump /
jump / jump / jump / jump

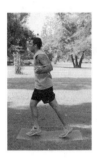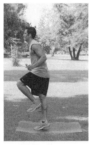

Running Man

lunge right / left knee up / lunge left / right knee up /
lunge right / left knee up / lunge left / right knee up

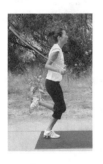

Run

run right / run left / run right / run left /
run right / run left / run right / run left

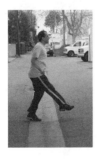

Step Kick Front

step left / kick right / step right / kick left /
step left / kick right / step right / kick left

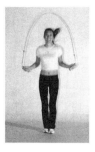 Heel Back

back right / center / back left / center /
back right / center / back left / center

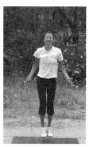 Boxer Shuffle

dig right / dig left / dig right / dig left /
dig right / dig left / dig right / dig left

Advanced Jump Combination 8

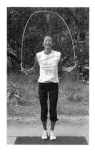 2 Foot Jump

jump / jump / jump / jump /
jump / jump / jump / jump

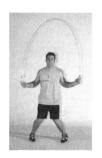 Straddle

out / center / out / center / out / center / out / center

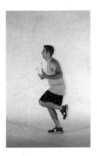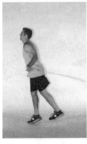

Step Kick Back

*step left / kick back right / step right / kick back left /
step left / kick back right / step right / kick back left*

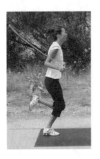

Run

*run right / run left / run right / run left /
run right / run left / run right / run left*

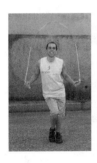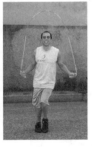

Alternating Foot

*hop right / hop left / hop right / hop left /
hop right / hop left / hop right / hop left*

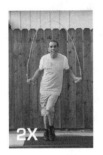

Alternating Foot, Double Bounce

*hop right / hop right / hop left / hop left /
hop right / hop right / hop left / hop left*

Advanced Jump Combination 9

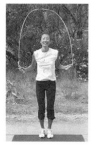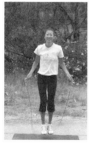

2 Foot Jump

jump / jump / jump / jump /
jump / jump / jump / jump

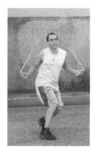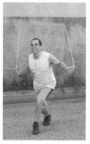

Touch Front and Back, right foot

touch front right / hop left /
touch back right / hop left /
touch front right / hop left /
touch back right / hop left

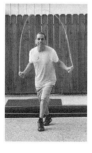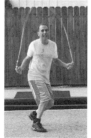

Touch Front and Back, left foot

touch front left / hop right /
touch back left / hop right /
touch front left / hop right /
touch back left / hop right

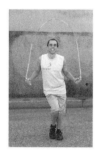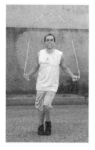

Alternating Foot

hop right / hop left / hop right / hop left /
hop right / hop left / hop right / hop left

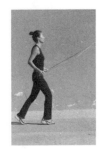

Lunge

lunge right / lunge left / lunge right / lunge left /
lunge right / lunge left / lunge right / lunge left

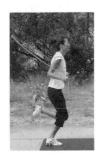

Run

run right / run left / run right / run left /
run right / run left / run right / run left

Advanced Jump Combination 10

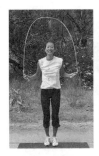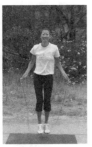

2 Foot Jump

jump / jump / jump / jump /
jump / jump / jump / jump

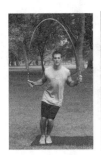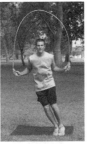

Slalom

right / left / right / left / right / left / right / left

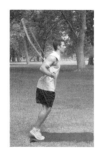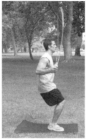

Front/Back

front / back / front / back / front / back / front / back

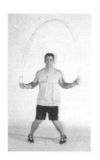

Straddle

out / center / out / center / out / center / out / center

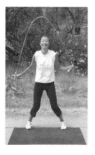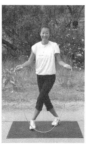

Foot Cross

straddle / cross / straddle / cross /
straddle / cross / straddle / cross

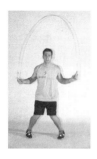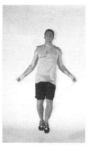

Heel Clicks

straddle, click / straddle, click / straddle, click /
straddle, click / straddle, click / straddle, click /
straddle, click / straddle, click

Advanced Jump Combination Bonus #1: Vertical Movement

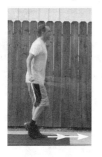

Alternating Foot, traveling forward

hop right / hop left / hop right / hop left /
hop right / hop left / hop right / hop left

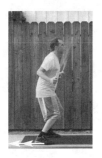

Straddle, traveling backward

out / center / out / center / out / center / out / center

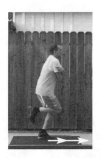

Run with Arm Crosses, traveling forward

cross arms, run right / uncross arms, run left /
cross arms, run right / uncross arms, run left /
cross arms, run right / uncross arms, run left /
cross arms, run right / uncross arms, run left

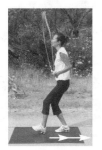

Boxer Shuffle, traveling backward

dig right / dig left / dig right / dig left /
dig right / dig left / dig right / dig left

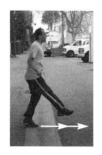

Step Kick Front, traveling forward

step left / kick right / step right / kick left /
step left / kick right / step right / kick left

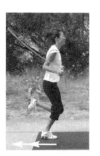

Heel Back, traveling backward

back right / center / back left / center /
back right / center / back left / center

Advanced Jump Combination Bonus #2: Increased Difficulty

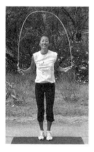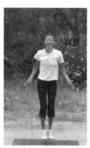

2 Foot Jump

jump / jump / jump / jump /
jump / jump / jump / jump

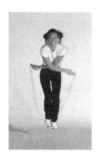

Crosses

cross / uncross / cross / uncross /
cross / uncross / cross / uncross

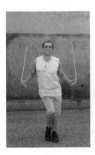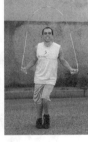

Alternating Foot

hop right / hop left / hop right / hop left /
hop right / hop left / hop right / hop left

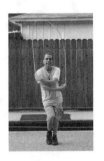

Alternating Foot with Arm Crosses

cross arms, hop right / uncross arms, hop left /
cross arms, hop right / uncross arms, hop left /
cross arms, hop right / uncross arms, hop left /
cross arms, hop right / uncross arms, hop left

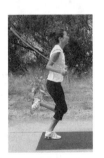

Run

run right / run left / run right / run left /
run right / run left / run right / run left

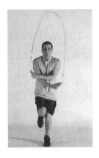

Run with Arm Crosses

cross arms, run right / uncross arms, run left /
cross arms, run right / uncross arms, run left /
cross arms, run right / uncross arms, run left /
cross arms, run right / uncross arms, run left

Chapter 18

Advanced RopeSport Workouts

(130–135 beats per minute; 45–60 minutes)

Use the following workouts on a weekly rotation. They should last you about a month. As your skill level improves, feel free to mix and match to fit your own unique style. Please note that the Advanced Workout Grid on pages 187–188 is meant to be used as a quick reference guide. The grid does not include Resting Moves between the jump sections or specific moves for the Stretches or Cooldowns. Please refer to the workout section below for a detailed list of the Stretches, Resting Moves, and Cooldowns.

Workout 1

Warm-up

- FreeStyle Rope Turns (1 minute)
- Figure 8 (4 × 8 counts)

- 2 Turns to Each Side (4 × 8 counts)
- Figure 8 (4 × 8 counts)
- Figure 8 High and Low (4 × 8 counts)
- Figure 8 (2 × 8 counts)
- Figure 8 Bouncing (4 × 8 counts)

- Figure 8 Bouncing, handles in the right hand only (2 × 8 counts)
- Figure 8 Bouncing, handles in the left hand only (2 × 8 counts)
- Figure 8 Bouncing (2 × 8 counts)
- 2 Foot Jump (4 × 8 counts)
- FreeStyle Jumping (20 seconds)
- Out of the rope
- Recover with Resting Moves (20 seconds)
- 2 Turns to Each Side (4 × 8 counts)
- Figure 8 (4 × 8 counts)
- Figure 8 Bouncing (4 × 8 counts)
- 2 Foot Jump (2 × 8 counts)
- Alternating Foot (4 × 8 counts)
- 2 Foot Jump (2 × 8 counts)
- FreeStyle Jumping (20 seconds)
- Out of the rope
- Recover with Resting Moves (20 seconds)
- Figure 8, right hand (8 counts)
- Figure 8, left hand (8 counts)

Warm-up Stretch (No Rope)

- Inhale 4 counts/exhale 4 counts (2 repetitions)
- Neck: head rotation (8 repetitions)
- Neck: head rolls (8 repetitions)
- Shoulders: shoulder circles, front and back (8 repetitions each direction)
- Triceps: arms across the body, right and left (holding 10 counts each side)
- Chest: hands clasped behind the back (holding 10 counts)
- Back: flex and extend (8 repetitions)
- Side and back: waist bend, right and left (holding 10 counts each side)
- Hamstrings: standing stretch, right and left (holding 10 counts each side)

- Groin and hips: runner's stretch, right and left (holding 10 counts each side)
- Hips and lower back: hip circles, right and left (8 repetitions each side)
- Ankles, feet, shins, and calves: roll front and back (8 repetitions)
- Calves: calf stretch, right and left (holding 10 counts each side)
- Shins: toe taps, right and left (16 repetitions each side)
- Ankles and feet: ankle circles, right and left (8 repetitions each side)

Jump 1

- FreeStyle Rope Turns (4 × 8 counts)
- Figure 8 (2 × 8 counts)
- 2 Turns to Each Side (2 × 8 counts)
- 2 Turns Step Touch (2 × 8 counts)
- Figure 8 (2 × 8 counts)
- Figure 8 Bouncing (2 × 8 counts)
- 2 Foot Jump (4 × 8 counts)
- Alternating Foot (4 × 8 counts)
- FreeStyle Jumping (30 seconds)
- Out of the rope
- Recover with Resting Moves (30 seconds to 1 minute)

Jump 2

- Figure 8 (2 × 8 counts)
- 2 Turns to Each Side (2 × 8 counts)
- 2 Turns Step Touch (2 × 8 counts)
- Figure 8 (2 × 8 counts)
- Figure 8 Bouncing (2 × 8 counts)
- 2 Foot Jump (5 × 8 counts)
- Boxer Shuffle (5 × 8 counts)
- FreeStyle Jumping (30 seconds)

- Out of the rope
- Recover with Resting Moves (30 seconds to 1 minute)

Sprint Jump 1

- Figure 8 (2 × 8 counts)
- 2 Turns to Each Side (2 × 8 counts)
- 2 Turns Step Touch (2 × 8 counts)
- Figure 8 (2 × 8 counts)
- Figure 8 Bouncing (2 × 8 counts)
- 2 Foot Jump Sprint (30 seconds)
- Out of the rope
- Recover with Resting Moves (30 seconds to 1 minute)

Sprint Jump 2

- Figure 8 (2 × 8 counts)
- 2 Turns to Each Side (2 × 8 counts)
- 2 Turns Step Touch (2 × 8 counts)
- Figure 8 (2 × 8 counts)
- Figure 8 Bouncing (2 × 8 counts)
- 2 Foot Jump Sprint (30 seconds)
- Out of the rope
- Recover with Resting Moves (30 seconds to 1 minute)

Recovery Jump

- Figure 8 (2 × 8 counts)
- 2 Turns to Each Side (2 × 8 counts)
- 2 Turns Step Touch (2 × 8 counts)
- Figure 8 (2 × 8 counts)
- Figure 8 Bouncing (2 × 8 counts)
- 2 Foot Jump (4 × 8 counts)
- Alternating Foot (4 × 8 counts)
- Out of the rope
- Recover with Resting Moves (30 seconds to 1 minute)

Jump 3

- Figure 8 (2 × 8 counts)
- 2 Turns to Each Side (2 × 8 counts)
- 2 Turns Step Touch (2 × 8 counts)
- Figure 8 (2 × 8 counts)
- Figure 8 Bouncing (2 × 8 counts)
- 2 Foot Jump (5 × 8 counts)
- Run (5 × 8 counts)
- FreeStyle Jumping (30 seconds)
- Out of the rope
- Recover with Resting Moves (30 seconds to 1 minute)

Jump 4

- Figure 8 (2 × 8 counts)
- 2 Turns to Each Side (2 × 8 counts)
- 2 Turns Step Touch (2 × 8 counts)
- Figure 8 (2 × 8 counts)
- Figure 8 Bouncing (2 × 8 counts)
- 2 Foot Jump (5 × 8 counts)
- Run, traveling forward (5 × 8 counts)
- FreeStyle Jumping (30 seconds)
- Out of the rope
- Recover with Resting Moves (30 seconds to 1 minute)

Combination

- Figure 8 (2 × 8 counts)
- 2 Turns to Each Side (2 × 8 counts)
- 2 Turns Step Touch (2 × 8 counts)
- Figure 8 (2 × 8 counts)
- Figure 8 Bouncing (2 × 8 counts)
- 2 Foot Jump (2 × 8 counts)
- Combination (2 to 4 sets)
  - 2 Foot Jump (8 counts)
  - Slalom (8 counts)

- Front/Back (8 counts)
- Lunge (8 counts)
- Run (8 counts)
- Alternating Foot (8 counts)
- Out of the rope
- Recover with Resting Moves (30 seconds to 1 minute)

Choreography (Long Jump): Around the World

- Figure 8 (2 × 8 counts)
- 2 Turns to Each Side (2 × 8 counts)
- 2 Turns Step Touch (2 × 8 counts)
- Figure 8 (2 × 8 counts)
- Figure 8 Bouncing (2 × 8 counts)
- 2 Foot Jump (2 × 8 counts)
- Around the World, right (4 × 8 counts)
  Turn around to the right, in a complete circle, jumping with the 2 Foot Jump, staying in one spot. Keep the jumps small and turn only a slight amount each jump to make sure not to get tangled in the rope. By the end of the jump you should be back where you started, completing a 360-degree turn.
- 2 Foot Jump (8 counts)
- Around the World, left (4 × 8 counts)

It's the same instructions as before, but this time you turn to the left.

- 2 Foot Jump (2 × 8 counts)
- Out of the rope
- Recover with Resting Moves (30 seconds to 1 minute)

Jump 5/Sprint Jump 3

- Figure 8 (2 × 8 counts)
- 2 Turns to Each Side (2 × 8 counts)

- 2 Turns Step Touch (2 × 8 counts)
- Figure 8 (2 × 8 counts)
- Figure 8 Bouncing (2 × 8 counts)
- 2 Foot Jump (8 × 8 counts)
- FreeStyle Sprint (20 seconds)
- Out of the rope
- Recover with Resting Moves (30 seconds to 1 minute)

Cooldown

- FreeStyle Rope Turns (1 minute)
- Figure 8 (2 × 8 counts)
- 2 Turns to Each Side (4 × 8 counts)
- 2 Turns Step Touch (4 × 8 counts)
- Figure 8 (2 × 8 counts)
- Figure 8 High and Low (4 × 8 counts)
- Figure 8 (2 × 8 counts)
- 2 Turns to Each Side (2 × 8 counts)
- 2 Turns Step Touch (2 × 8 counts)
- Figure 8 (2 × 8 counts)
- Figure 8, right hand (8 counts)
- Figure 8, left hand (8 counts)

Strength

- Legs and butt (3 to 4 sets)
- Squats (8 to 12 repetitions)
- Double-time pulsing squats (16 to 24 repetitions)
  Be sure to take a short break between squat sets.

Cooldown Stretch: Supine, Seated, and Standing (No Rope)

- Glutes and lower back: supine knee to chest, right and left side (holding 10 seconds each side)

- Glutes and lower back: twist to side, right and left side (holding 10 seconds each side)
- Placing hands behind the thighs, slowly roll yourself up to a seated position.
- Groin and hips: seated butterfly (hold 20 seconds)
- Hamstrings and calves: seated legs extended (holding 20 seconds)
- Groin, hips, and hamstrings: seated straddle (holding 20 seconds)
- Slowly bring yourself off the floor to a standing position.
- Neck: head rolls (8 repetitions)
- Shoulders: shoulder circles, front and back (8 repetitions each direction)
- Triceps: arms cocked behind head, right and left (holding 10 counts each side)
- Chest: hands clasped behind the back (holding 10 counts)
- Side and back: waist bend, right and left (holding 10 counts each side)
- Hips and lower back: hip circles, right and left (8 repetitions each direction)
- Hamstrings: standing stretch, right and left (holding 10 counts each side)
- Calves: calf stretch, right and left (holding 10 counts each side)
- Ankles and feet: ankle circles, right and left (8 repetitions each side)
- Inhale 4 counts/exhale 4 counts (2 repetitions)

Workout 2

Warm-up

- FreeStyle Rope Turns (1 minute)
- Figure 8 (4 × 8 counts)

- 2 Turns to Each Side (4 × 8 counts)
- Figure 8 (4 × 8 counts)
- Figure 8 High and Low (4 × 8 counts)
- Figure 8 (2 × 8 counts)
- Figure 8 Bouncing (4 × 8 counts)
- Figure 8 Bouncing, handles in the right hand only (2 × 8 counts)
- Figure 8 Bouncing, handles in the left hand only (2 × 8 counts)
- Figure 8 Bouncing (2 × 8 counts)
- 2 Foot Jump (4 × 8 counts)
- FreeStyle Jumping (20 seconds)
- Out of the rope
- Recover with Resting Moves (20 seconds)
- 2 Turns to Each Side (4 × 8 counts)
- Figure 8 (4 × 8 counts)
- Figure 8 Bouncing (4 × 8 counts)
- 2 Foot Jump (2 × 8 counts)
- Alternating Foot (4 × 8 counts)
- 2 Foot Jump (2 × 8 counts)
- FreeStyle Jumping (20 seconds)
- Out of the rope
- Recover with Resting Moves (20 seconds)
- Figure 8, right hand (8 counts)
- Figure 8, left hand (8 counts)

Warm-up Stretch (No Rope)

- Inhale 4 counts/exhale 4 counts (2 repetitions)
- Neck: head rotation (8 repetitions)
- Neck: head rolls (8 repetitions)
- Shoulders: shoulder circles, front and back (8 repetitions each direction)
- Triceps: arms across the body, right and left (holding 10 counts each side)
- Chest: hands clasped behind the back (holding 10 counts)

- Back: flex and extend (8 repetitions)
- Side and back: waist bend, right and left (holding 10 counts each side)
- Hamstrings: standing stretch, right and left (holding 10 counts each side)
- Groin and hips: runner's stretch, right and left (holding 10 counts each side)
- Hips and lower back: hip circles, right and left (8 repetitions each side)
- Ankles, feet, shins, and calves: roll front and back (8 repetitions)
- Calves: calf stretch, right and left (holding 10 counts each side)
- Shins: toe taps, right and left (16 repetitions each side)
- Ankles and feet: ankle circles, right and left (8 repetitions each side)

Jump 1

- FreeStyle Rope Turns (4 × 8 counts)
- Figure 8 (2 × 8 counts)
- 2 Turns to Each Side (2 × 8 counts)
- 2 Turns Step Touch (2 × 8 counts)
- Figure 8 (2 × 8 counts)
- Figure 8 Bouncing (2 × 8 counts)
- 2 Foot Jump (4 × 8 counts)
- Boxer Shuffle (4 × 8 counts)
- FreeStyle Jumping (30 seconds)
- Out of the rope
- Recover with Resting Moves (30 seconds to 1 minute)

Jump 2

- Figure 8 (2 × 8 counts)
- 2 Turns to Each Side (2 × 8 counts)
- 2 Turns Step Touch (2 × 8 counts)

- Figure 8 (2 × 8 counts)
- Figure 8 Bouncing (2 × 8 counts)
- 2 Foot Jump (5 × 8 counts)
- Run (5 × 8 counts)
- FreeStyle Jumping (30 seconds)
- Out of the rope
- Recover with Resting Moves (30 seconds to 1 minute)

Sprint Jump 1

- Figure 8 (2 × 8 counts)
- 2 Turns to Each Side (2 × 8 counts)
- 2 Turns Step Touch (2 × 8 counts)
- Figure 8 (2 × 8 counts)
- Figure 8 Bouncing (2 × 8 counts)
- 2 Foot Jump Sprint (15 seconds)
- Run Sprint (15 seconds)
- Out of the rope
- Recover with Resting Moves (30 seconds to 1 minute)

Sprint Jump 2

- Figure 8 (2 × 8 counts)
- 2 Turns to Each Side (2 × 8 counts)
- 2 Turns Step Touch (2 × 8 counts)
- Figure 8 (2 × 8 counts)
- Figure 8 Bouncing (2 × 8 counts)
- 2 Foot Jump Sprint (15 seconds)
- Alternating Foot Sprint (15 seconds)
- Out of the rope
- Recover with Resting Moves (30 seconds to 1 minute)

Recovery Jump

- Figure 8 (2 × 8 counts)
- 2 Turns to Each Side (2 × 8 counts)
- 2 Turns Step Touch (2 × 8 counts)

- Figure 8 (2 × 8 counts)
- Figure 8 Bouncing (2 × 8 counts)
- 2 Foot Jump (4 × 8 counts)
- Boxer Shuffle (4 × 8 counts)
- Out of the rope
- Recover with Resting Moves (30 seconds to 1 minute)

Jump 3

- Figure 8 (2 × 8 counts)
- 2 Turns to Each Side (2 × 8 counts)
- 2 Turns Step Touch (2 × 8 counts)
- Figure 8 (2 × 8 counts)
- Figure 8 Bouncing (2 × 8 counts)
- 2 Foot Jump (5 × 8 counts)
- Slalom (5 × 8 counts)
- FreeStyle Jumping (30 seconds)
- Out of the rope
- Recover with Resting Moves (30 seconds to 1 minute)

Jump 4

- Figure 8 (2 × 8 counts)
- 2 Turns to Each Side (2 × 8 counts)
- 2 Turns Step Touch (2 × 8 counts)
- Figure 8 (2 × 8 counts)
- Figure 8 Bouncing (2 × 8 counts)
- 2 Foot Jump (5 × 8 counts)
- Straddle (5 × 8 counts)
- FreeStyle Jumping (30 seconds)
- Out of the rope
- Recover with Resting Moves (30 seconds to 1 minute)

Combination

- Figure 8 (2 × 8 counts)
- 2 Turns to Each Side (2 × 8 counts)

- 2 Turns Step Touch (2 × 8 counts)
- Figure 8 (2 × 8 counts)
- Figure 8 Bouncing (2 × 8 counts)
- 2 Foot Jump (2 × 8 counts)
- Combination (2 to 4 sets)
  - 2 Foot Jump (8 counts)
  - Run (8 counts)
  - Run, Double Bounce (8 counts)
  - Boxer Shuffle (8 counts)
  - Boxer Shuffle, Double Bounce (8 counts)
  - Alternating Foot (8 counts)
- Out of the rope
- Recover with Resting Moves (30 seconds to 1 minute)

Choreography (Long Jump): Around the World II

- Figure 8 (2 × 8 counts)
- 2 Turns to Each Side (2 × 8 counts)
- 2 Turns Step Touch (2 × 8 counts)
- Figure 8 (2 × 8 counts)
- Figure 8 Bouncing (2 × 8 counts)
- 2 Foot Jump (2 × 8 counts)
- Around the World II, right (4 × 8 counts)
  - V Jump (jumping left, center, right, center)
  - 2 Foot Jump (turning right 90 degrees on each 4 counts)

  Repeat four times: front, right side, back, left side. You should end back where you started—facing the front.
- 2 Foot Jump (8 counts)
- Around the World II, left (4 × 8 counts)
  - V Jump (jumping right, center, left, center)

- 2 Foot Jump (turning left 90 degrees on each 4 counts)

Repeat four times: front, left side, back, right side. You should end back where you started—facing the front.

- Out of the rope
- Recover with Resting Moves (30 seconds to 1 minute)

Jump 5/Sprint Jump 3

- Figure 8 (2 × 8 counts)
- 2 Turns to Each Side (2 × 8 counts)
- 2 Turns Step Touch (2 × 8 counts)
- Figure 8 (2 × 8 counts)
- Figure 8 Bouncing (2 × 8 counts)
- 2 Foot Jump (5 × 8 counts)
- Alternating Foot (5 × 8 counts)
- FreeStyle Sprint (20 seconds)
- Out of the rope
- Recover with Resting Moves (30 seconds to 1 minute)

Cooldown

- FreeStyle Rope Turns (1 minute)
- Figure 8 (2 × 8 counts)
- 2 Turns to Each Side (4 × 8 counts)
- 2 Turns Step Touch (4 × 8 counts)
- Figure 8 (2 × 8 counts)
- Figure 8 High and Low (4 × 8 counts)
- Figure 8 (2 × 8 counts)
- 2 Turns to Each Side (2 × 8 counts)
- 2 Turns Step Touch (2 × 8 counts)
- Figure 8 (2 × 8 counts)
- Figure 8, right hand (8 counts)
- Figure 8, left hand (8 counts)

Strength

- Abdominals (3 to 4 sets)
  - Crunches (8 to 12 repetitions)
  - Rotation crunches (16 to 24 repetitions)

Be sure to take a short break between crunch sets.

Cooldown Stretch: Supine, Seated, and Standing (No Rope)

- Glutes and lower back: supine knee to chest, right and left side (holding 10 seconds each side)
- Glutes and lower back: twist to side, right and left side (holding 10 seconds each side)
- Placing hands behind the thighs, slowly roll yourself up to a seated position.
- Groin and hips: seated butterfly (holding 20 seconds)
- Hamstrings and calves: seated legs extended (holding 20 seconds)
- Groin, hips, and hamstrings: seated straddle (holding 20 seconds)
- Slowly bring yourself off the floor to a standing position.
- Neck: head rolls (8 repetitions)
- Shoulders: shoulder circles, front and back (8 repetitions each direction)
- Triceps: arms cocked behind head, right and left (holding 10 counts each side)
- Chest: hands clasped behind the back (holding 10 counts)
- Side and back: waist bend, right and left (holding 10 counts each side)
- Hips and lower back: hip circles, right and left (8 repetitions each direction)

- Hamstrings: standing stretch, right and left (holding 10 counts each side)
- Calves: calf stretch, right and left (holding 10 counts each side)
- Ankles and feet: ankle circles, right and left (8 repetitions each side)
- Inhale 4 counts/exhale 4 counts (2 repetitions)

Workout 3

Warm-up

- FreeStyle Rope Turns (1 minute)
- Figure 8 (4 × 8 counts)
- 2 Turns to Each Side (4 × 8 counts)
- Figure 8 (4 × 8 counts)
- Figure 8 High and Low (4 × 8 counts)
- Figure 8 (2 × 8 counts)
- Figure 8 Bouncing (4 × 8 counts)
- Figure 8 Bouncing, handles in the right hand only (2 × 8 counts)
- Figure 8 Bouncing, handles in the left hand only (2 × 8 counts)
- Figure 8 Bouncing (2 × 8 counts)
- 2 Foot Jump (4 × 8 counts)
- FreeStyle Jumping (20 seconds)
- Out of the rope
- Recover with Resting Moves (20 seconds)
- 2 Turns to Each Side (4 × 8 counts)
- Figure 8 (4 × 8 counts)
- Figure 8 Bouncing (4 × 8 counts)
- 2 Foot Jump (2 × 8 counts)
- Alternating Foot (4 × 8 counts)
- 2 Foot Jump (2 × 8 counts)
- FreeStyle Jumping (20 seconds)
- Out of the rope

- Recover with Resting Moves (20 seconds)
- Figure 8, right hand (8 counts)
- Figure 8, left hand (8 counts)

Warm-up Stretch (No Rope)

- Inhale 4 counts/exhale 4 counts (2 repetitions)
- Neck: head rotation (8 repetitions)
- Neck: head rolls (8 repetitions)
- Shoulders: shoulder circles, front and back (8 repetitions each direction)
- Triceps: arms across the body, right and left (holding 10 counts each side)
- Chest: hands clasped behind the back (holding 10 counts)
- Back: flex and extend (8 repetitions)
- Side and back: waist bend, right and left (holding 10 counts each side)
- Hamstrings: standing stretch, right and left (holding 10 counts each side)
- Groin and hips: runner's stretch, right and left (holding 10 counts each side)
- Hips and lower back: hip circles, right and left (8 repetitions each side)
- Ankles, feet, shins, and calves: roll front and back (8 repetitions)
- Calves: calf stretch, right and left (holding 10 counts each side)
- Shins: toe taps, right and left (16 repetitions each side)
- Ankles and feet: ankle circles, right and left (8 repetitions each side)

Jump 1

- FreeStyle Rope Turns (4 × 8 counts)
- Figure 8 (2 × 8 counts)
- 2 Turns to Each Side (2 × 8 counts)

- 2 Turns Step Touch (2 × 8 counts)
- Figure 8 (2 × 8 counts)
- Figure 8 Bouncing (2 × 8 counts)
- 2 Foot Jump (4 × 8 counts)
- Run (4 × 8 counts)
- FreeStyle Jumping (30 seconds)
- Out of the rope
- Recover with Resting Moves (30 seconds to 1 minute)

Jump 2

- Figure 8 (2 × 8 counts)
- 2 Turns to Each Side (2 × 8 counts)
- 2 Turns Step Touch (2 × 8 counts)
- Figure 8 (2 × 8 counts)
- Figure 8 Bouncing (2 × 8 counts)
- 2 Foot Jump (5 × 8 counts)
- Slalom (5 × 8 counts)
- FreeStyle Jumping (30 seconds)
- Out of the rope
- Recover with Resting Moves (30 seconds to 1 minute)

Sprint Jump 1

- Figure 8 (2 × 8 counts)
- 2 Turns to Each Side (2 × 8 counts)
- 2 Turns Step Touch (2 × 8 counts)
- Figure 8 (2 × 8 counts)
- Figure 8 Bouncing (2 × 8 counts)
- 2 Foot Jump Sprint (15 seconds)
- Boxer Shuffle Sprint (15 seconds)
- Out of the rope
- Recover with Resting Moves (30 seconds to 1 minute)

Sprint Jump 2

- Figure 8 (2 × 8 counts)
- 2 Turns to Each Side (2 × 8 counts)
- 2 Turns Step Touch (2 × 8 counts)
- Figure 8 (2 × 8 counts)
- Figure 8 Bouncing (2 × 8 counts)
- 2 Foot Jump Sprint (15 seconds)
- Straddle (15 seconds)
- Out of the rope
- Recover with Resting Moves (30 seconds to 1 minute)

Recovery Jump

- Figure 8 (2 × 8 counts)
- 2 Turns to Each Side (2 × 8 counts)
- 2 Turns Step Touch (2 × 8 counts)
- Figure 8 (2 × 8 counts)
- Figure 8 Bouncing (2 × 8 counts)
- 2 Foot Jump (4 × 8 counts)
- Run (4 × 8 counts)
- Out of the rope
- Recover with Resting Moves (30 seconds to 1 minute)

Jump 3

- Figure 8 (2 × 8 counts)
- 2 Turns to Each Side (2 × 8 counts)
- 2 Turns Step Touch (2 × 8 counts)
- Figure 8 (2 × 8 counts)
- Figure 8 Bouncing (2 × 8 counts)
- 2 Foot Jump (5 × 8 counts)
- Front/Back (5 × 8 counts)
- FreeStyle Jumping (30 seconds)
- Out of the rope
- Recover with Resting Moves (30 seconds to 1 minute)

Jump 4

- Figure 8 (2 × 8 counts)
- 2 Turns to Each Side (2 × 8 counts)
- 2 Turns Step Touch (2 × 8 counts)
- Figure 8 (2 × 8 counts)
- Figure 8 Bouncing (2 × 8 counts)
- 2 Foot Jump (5 × 8 counts)
- Lunge (5 × 8 counts)
- FreeStyle Jumping (30 seconds)
- Out of the rope
- Recover with Resting Moves (30 seconds to 1 minute)

Combination

- Figure 8 (2 × 8 counts)
- 2 Turns to Each Side (2 × 8 counts)
- 2 Turns Step Touch (2 × 8 counts)
- Figure 8 (2 × 8 counts)
- Figure 8 Bouncing (2 × 8 counts)
- 2 Foot Jump (2 × 8 counts)
- Combination (2 to 4 sets)
  - 2 Foot Jump (8 counts)
  - Alternating Foot (8 counts)
  - Alternating Foot/Double Bounce (8 counts)
  - Slalom (8 counts)
  - Straddle (8 counts)
  - Alternating Foot (8 counts)
- Out of the rope
- Recover with Resting Moves (30 seconds to 1 minute)

Choreography (Long Jump): The Rope Run

- Figure 8 (2 × 8 counts)
- 2 Turns to Each Side (2 × 8 counts)

- 2 Turns Step Touch (2 × 8 counts)
- Figure 8 (2 × 8 counts)
- Figure 8 Bouncing (2 × 8 counts)
- 2 Foot Jump (2 × 8 counts)
- The Rope Run (13 × 8 counts)

  This choreography alternates going in the rope with the 2 Foot Jump for 8 counts, and out of the rope with the Figure 8 Bouncing for 8 counts.

  - 2 Foot Jump (2 × 8 counts)
  - Figure 8 Bouncing (2 × 8 counts)
  - 2 Foot Jump (8 counts)
  - Figure 8 Bouncing (8 counts)
  - 2 Foot Jump (8 counts)
  - Figure 8 Bouncing (8 counts)
  - 2 Foot Jump (8 counts)
  - Figure 8 Bouncing (8 counts)
  - 2 Foot Jump (4 counts)
  - Figure 8 Bouncing (4 counts)
  - 2 Foot Jump (4 counts)
  - Figure 8 Bouncing (4 counts)
  - 2 Foot Jump (4 counts)
  - Figure 8 Bouncing (4 counts)
- 2 Foot Jump (2 × 8 counts)
- Out of the rope
- Recover with Resting Moves (30 seconds to 1 minute)

Jump 5/Sprint Jump 3

- Figure 8 (2 × 8 counts)
- 2 Turns to Each Side (2 × 8 counts)
- 2 Turns Step Touch (2 × 8 counts)
- Figure 8 (2 × 8 counts)
- Figure 8 Bouncing (2 × 8 counts)
- 2 Foot Jump (5 × 8 counts)
- Run (5 × 8 counts)

- FreeStyle Sprint (20 seconds)
- Out of the rope
- Recover with Resting Moves (30 seconds to 1 minute)

Cooldown

- FreeStyle Rope Turns (1 minute)
- Figure 8 (2 × 8 counts)
- 2 Turns to Each Side (4 × 8 counts)
- 2 Turns Step Touch (4 × 8 counts)
- Figure 8 (2 × 8 counts)
- Figure 8 High and Low (4 × 8 counts)
- Figure 8 (2 × 8 counts)
- 2 Turns to Each Side (2 × 8 counts)
- 2 Turns Step Touch (2 × 8 counts)
- Figure 8 (2 × 8 counts)
- Figure 8, right hand (8 counts)
- Figure 8, left hand (8 counts)

Strength

- Chest and arms (3 to 4 sets)
  - Double-time push-ups (5 repetitions)
  - Push-ups (10 repetitions)
  Be sure to take a short break between push-up sets.

Cooldown Stretch: Supine, Seated, and Standing (No Rope)

- Glutes and lower back: supine knee to chest, right and left side (holding 10 seconds each side)
- Glutes and lower back: twist to side, right and left side (holding 10 seconds each side)
- Placing hands behind the thighs, slowly roll yourself up to a seated position.

- Groin and hips: seated butterfly (holding 20 seconds)
- Hamstrings and calves: seated legs extended (holding 20 seconds)
- Groin, hips, and hamstrings: seated straddle (holding 20 seconds)
- Slowly bring yourself off the floor to a standing position.
- Neck: head rolls (8 repetitions)
- Shoulders: shoulder circles, front and back (8 repetitions each direction)
- Triceps: arms cocked behind head, right and left (holding 10 counts each side)
- Chest: hands clasped behind the back (holding 10 counts)
- Side and back: waist bend, right and left (holding 10 counts each side)
- Hips and lower back: hip circles, right and left (8 repetitions each direction)
- Hamstrings: standing stretch, right and left (holding 10 counts each side)
- Calves: calf stretch, right and left (holding 10 counts each side)
- Ankles and feet: ankle circles, right and left (8 repetitions each side)
- Inhale 4 counts/exhale 4 counts (2 repetitions)

Workout 4

Warm-up

- FreeStyle Rope Turns (1 minute)
- Figure 8 (4 × 8 counts)
- 2 Turns to Each Side (4 × 8 counts)
- Figure 8 (4 × 8 counts)
- Figure 8 High and Low (4 × 8 counts)
- Figure 8 (2 × 8 counts)

- Figure 8 Bouncing (4 × 8 counts)
- Figure 8 Bouncing, handles in the right hand only (2 × 8 counts)
- Figure 8 Bouncing, handles in the left hand only (2 × 8 counts)
- Figure 8 Bouncing (2 × 8 counts)
- 2 Foot Jump (4 × 8 counts)
- FreeStyle Jumping (20 seconds)
- Out of the rope
- Recover with Resting Moves (20 seconds)
- 2 Turns to Each Side (4 × 8 counts)
- Figure 8 (4 × 8 counts)
- Figure 8 Bouncing (4 × 8 counts)
- 2 Foot Jump (2 × 8 counts)
- Alternating Foot (4 × 8 counts)
- 2 Foot Jump (2 × 8 counts)
- FreeStyle Jumping (20 seconds)
- Out of the rope
- Recover with Resting Moves (20 seconds)
- Figure 8, right hand (8 counts)
- Figure 8, left hand (8 counts)

Warm-up Stretch (No Rope)

- Inhale 4 counts/exhale 4 counts (2 repetitions)
- Neck: head rotation (8 repetitions)
- Neck: head rolls (8 repetitions)
- Shoulders: shoulder circles, front and back (8 repetitions each direction)
- Triceps: arms across the body, right and left (holding 10 counts each side)
- Chest: hands clasped behind the back (holding 10 counts)
- Back: flex and extend (8 repetitions)
- Side and back: waist bend, right and left (holding 10 counts each side)

- Hamstrings: standing stretch, right and left (holding 10 counts each side)
- Groin and hips: runner's stretch, right and left (holding 10 counts each side)
- Hips and lower back: hip circles, right and left (8 repetitions each side)
- Ankles, feet, shins, and calves: roll front and back (8 repetitions)
- Calves: calf stretch, right and left (holding 10 counts each side)
- Shins: toe taps, right and left (16 repetitions each side)
- Ankles and feet: ankle circles, right and left (8 repetitions each side)

Jump 1

- FreeStyle Rope Turns (4 × 8 counts)
- Figure 8 (2 × 8 counts)
- 2 Turns to Each Side (2 × 8 counts)
- 2 Turns Step Touch (2 × 8 counts)
- Figure 8 (2 × 8 counts)
- Figure 8 Bouncing (2 × 8 counts)
- 2 Foot Jump (4 × 8 counts)
- Lunge (4 × 8 counts)
- FreeStyle Jumping (30 seconds)
- Out of the rope
- Recover with Resting Moves (30 seconds to 1 minute)

Jump 2

- Figure 8 (2 × 8 counts)
- 2 Turns to Each Side (2 × 8 counts)
- 2 Turns Step Touch (2 × 8 counts)
- Figure 8 (2 × 8 counts)
- Figure 8 Bouncing (2 × 8 counts)
- 2 Foot Jump (5 × 8 counts)

- Front/Back (5 × 8 counts)
- FreeStyle Jumping (30 seconds)
- Out of the rope
- Recover with Resting Moves (30 seconds to 1 minute)

Sprint Jump 1

- Figure 8 (2 × 8 counts)
- 2 Turns to Each Side (2 × 8 counts)
- 2 Turns Step Touch (2 × 8 counts)
- Figure 8 (2 × 8 counts)
- Figure 8 Bouncing (2 × 8 counts)
- 2 Foot Jump Sprint (15 seconds)
- Slalom Sprint (15 seconds)
- Out of the rope
- Recover with Resting Moves (30 seconds to 1 minute)

Sprint Jump 2

- Figure 8 (2 × 8 counts)
- 2 Turns to Each Side (2 × 8 counts)
- 2 Turns Step Touch (2 × 8 counts)
- Figure 8 (2 × 8 counts)
- Figure 8 Bouncing (2 × 8 counts)
- 2 Foot Jump Sprint (15 seconds)
- Run Sprint (15 seconds)
- Out of the rope
- Recover with Resting Moves (30 seconds to 1 minute)

Recovery Jump

- Figure 8 (2 × 8 counts)
- 2 Turns to Each Side (2 × 8 counts)
- 2 Turns Step Touch (2 × 8 counts)
- Figure 8 (2 × 8 counts)
- Figure 8 Bouncing (2 × 8 counts)

- 2 Foot Jump (4 × 8 counts)
- Slalom (4 × 8 counts)
- Out of the rope
- Recover with Resting Moves (30 seconds to 1 minute)

Jump 3

- Figure 8 (2 × 8 counts)
- 2 Turns to Each Side (2 × 8 counts)
- 2 Turns Step Touch (2 × 8 counts)
- Figure 8 (2 × 8 counts)
- Figure 8 Bouncing (2 × 8 counts)
- 2 Foot Jump (5 × 8 counts)
- Straddle (5 × 8 counts)
- FreeStyle Jumping (30 seconds)
- Out of the rope
- Recover with Resting Moves (30 seconds to 1 minute)

Jump 4

- Figure 8 (2 × 8 counts)
- 2 Turns to Each Side (2 × 8 counts)
- 2 Turns Step Touch (2 × 8 counts)
- Figure 8 (2 × 8 counts)
- Figure 8 Bouncing (2 × 8 counts)
- 2 Foot Jump (5 × 8 counts)
- V Jump (5 × 8 counts)
- FreeStyle Jumping (30 seconds)
- Out of the rope
- Recover with Resting Moves (30 seconds to 1 minute)

Combination

- Figure 8 (2 × 8 counts)
- 2 Turns to Each Side (2 × 8 counts)
- 2 Turns Step Touch (2 × 8 counts)

- Figure 8 (2 × 8 counts)
- Figure 8 Bouncing (2 × 8 counts)
- 2 Foot Jump (2 × 8 counts)
- Combination (2 to 4 sets)
  - 2 Foot Jump (8 counts)
  - Slalom (8 counts)
  - V Jump (8 counts)
  - Lunge (8 counts)
  - Run (8 counts)
  - Alternating Foot (8 counts)
- Out of the rope
- Recover with Resting Moves (30 seconds to 1 minute)

Choreography (Long Jump): The Run and Hop

- Figure 8 (2 × 8 counts)
- 2 Turns to Each Side (2 × 8 counts)
- 2 Turns Step Touch (2 × 8 counts)
- Figure 8 (2 × 8 counts)
- Figure 8 Bouncing (2 × 8 counts)
- 2 Foot Jump (2 × 8 counts)
- The Run and Hop (14 × 8 counts)
  - Run, traveling forward (2 × 8 counts)
  - 2 Foot Jump, traveling backward (2 × 8 counts)
  - Run, traveling forward (2 × 8 counts)
  - 2 Foot Jump, traveling backward (2 × 8 counts)
  - Run, traveling forward (8 counts)
  - 2 Foot Jump, traveling backward (8 counts)
  - Run, traveling forward (8 counts)
  - 2 Foot Jump, traveling backward (8 counts)
  - Run, traveling forward (8 counts)
  - 2 Foot Jump, traveling backward (8 counts)
- 2 Foot Jump (2 × 8 counts)

- Out of the rope
- Recover with Resting Moves (30 seconds to 1 minute)

Jump 5/Sprint Jump 3

- Figure 8 (2 × 8 counts)
- 2 Turns to Each Side (2 × 8 counts)
- 2 Turns Step Touch (2 × 8 counts)
- Figure 8 (2 × 8 counts)
- Figure 8 Bouncing (2 × 8 counts)
- 2 Foot Jump (5 × 8 counts)
- Slalom (5 × 8 counts)
- FreeStyle Sprint (20 seconds)
- Out of the rope
- Recover with Resting Moves (30 seconds to 1 minute)

Cooldown

- FreeStyle Rope Turns (1 minute)
- Figure 8 (2 × 8 counts)
- 2 Turns to Each Side (4 × 8 counts)
- 2 Turns Step Touch (4 × 8 counts)
- Figure 8 (2 × 8 counts)
- Figure 8 High and Low (4 × 8 counts)
- Figure 8 (2 × 8 counts)
- 2 Turns to Each Side (2 × 8 counts)
- 2 Turns Step Touch (2 × 8 counts)
- Figure 8 (2 × 8 counts)
- Figure 8, right hand (8 counts)
- Figure 8, left hand (8 counts)

Strength

- Legs and butt (3 to 4 sets)
  - Alternating Lunges (16 to 24 repetitions)
  - Same-Side Lunges, right and left side (8 to 12 repetitions each side)

Be sure to take a short break between squat sets.

Cooldown Stretch: Supine, Seated, and Standing (No Rope)

- Glutes and lower back: supine knee to chest, right and left side (holding 10 seconds each side)
- Glutes and lower back: twist to side, right and left side (holding 10 seconds each side)
- Placing hands behind the thighs, slowly roll yourself up to a seated position.
- Groin and hips: seated butterfly (hold 20 seconds)
- Hamstrings and calves: seated legs extended (holding 20 seconds)
- Groin, hips, and hamstrings: seated straddle (holding 20 seconds)
- Slowly bring yourself off the floor to a standing position.
- Neck: head rolls (8 repetitions)

- Shoulders: shoulder circles, front and back (8 repetitions each direction)
- Triceps: arms cocked behind head, right and left (holding 10 counts each side)
- Chest: hands clasped behind the back (holding 10 counts)
- Side and back: waist bend, right and left (holding 10 counts each side)
- Hips and lower back: hip circles, right and left (8 repetitions each direction)
- Hamstrings: standing stretch, right and left (holding 10 counts each side)
- Calves: calf stretch, right and left (holding 10 counts each side)
- Ankles and feet: ankle circles, right and left (8 repetitions each side)
- Inhale 4 counts/exhale 4 counts (2 repetitions)

Advanced Workout Grid

Advanced Workout 1	Advanced Workout 2	Advanced Workout 3	Advanced Workout 4
Warm-up	Warm-up	Warm-up	Warm-up
Warm-up Stretch	Warm-up Stretch	Warm-up Stretch	Warm-up Stretch
Jump 1 2 Foot Jump Alternating Foot FreeStyle	**Jump 1** 2 Foot Jump Boxer Shuffle FreeStyle	**Jump 1** 2 Foot Jump Run FreeStyle	**Jump 1** 2 Foot Jump Lunge FreeStyle
Jump 2 2 Foot Jump Boxer Shuffle FreeStyle	**Jump 2** 2 Foot Jump Run FreeStyle	**Jump 2** 2 Foot Jump Slalom FreeStyle	**Jump 2** 2 Foot Jump Front/Back FreeStyle
Sprint Jump 1 2 Foot Jump	**Sprint Jump 1** 2 Foot Jump Run	**Sprint Jump 1** 2 Foot Jump Boxer Shuffle	**Sprint Jump 1** 2 Foot Jump Slalom

Advanced Workout 1	Advanced Workout 2	Advanced Workout 3	Advanced Workout 4
Sprint Jump 2 2 Foot Jump	**Sprint Jump 2** 2 Foot Jump Alternating Foot	**Sprint Jump 2** 2 Foot Jump Straddle	**Sprint Jump 2** 2 Foot Jump Run
Recovery Jump 2 Foot Jump Alternating Foot	**Recovery Jump** 2 Foot Jump Boxer Shuffle	**Recovery Jump** 2 Foot Jump Run	**Recovery Jump** 2 Foot Jump Slalom
Jump 3 2 Foot Jump Run FreeStyle	**Jump 3** 2 Foot Jump Slalom FreeStyle	**Jump 3** 2 Foot Jump Front/Back FreeStyle	**Jump 3** 2 Foot Jump Straddle FreeStyle
Jump 4 2 Foot Jump Run with Vertical Movement FreeStyle	**Jump 4** 2 Foot Jump Straddle FreeStyle	**Jump 4** 2 Foot Jump Lunge FreeStyle	**Jump 4** 2 Foot Jump V Jump FreeStyle
Combination 2 Foot Jump Slalom Front/Back Lunge Run Alternating Foot	**Combination** 2 Foot Jump Run Run/Double Bounce Boxer Shuffle Boxer Shuffle/ Double Bounce Alternating Foot	**Combination** 2 Foot Jump Alternating Foot Alternating Foot/ Double Bounce Slalom Straddle Alternating Foot	**Combination** 2 Foot Jump Slalom V Jump Lunge Run Alternating Foot
Choreography (Long Jump): Around the World	**Choreography (Long Jump): Around theWorld**	**Choreography (Long Jump): The Rope Run**	**Choreography (Long Jump): The Run and Hop**
Jump 5/Sprint Jump 3 2 Foot Jump FreeStyle Sprint (20)	**Jump 5/Sprint Jump 3** 2 Foot Jump Alternating Foot FreeStyle Sprint (20)	**Jump 5/Sprint Jump 3** 2 Foot Jump Run FreeStyle Sprint (20)	**Jump 5/Sprint Jump 3** 2 Foot Jump Slalom FreeStyle Sprint (20)
Cooldown	**Cooldown**	**Cooldown**	**Cooldown**
Strength Squats Single/Double Time	**Strength** Crunches Basic and Rotating	**Strength** Push-ups Single/Double Time	**Strength** Alternating and Same-Side Lunges
Cooldown Stretch	**Cooldown Stretch**	**Cooldown Stretch**	**Cooldown Stretch**

Chapter 19

Extreme Jumps

If you can master just a few of the following Extreme Jumps, you'll be in the top 1 percent of people who have ever held a jump rope in their hands. Most of these Extreme Jumps aren't learned overnight and take a lot of patience to master. Some of them require speed and power, others require agility and coordination, and others a combination of both. As with any new jump that's difficult to learn, I suggest practicing a specific jump for no more than five minutes and then moving on to something else. Give yourself a break and only practice the same jump later in your workout or during your next workout. This is also the perfect time to utilize the Three-Step Breakdown and to consider using your speed rope for maximum rotation speed.

Some of these Extreme Jumps, many of which are quite intricate, can be a little tricky to describe verbally or with still photos that only capture part of the jump. If you are interested in more detailed information, you should consider reviewing our RopeSport Extreme DVD, which would help clarify any questions you have regarding how a specific jump is done.

Matador

The Matador is a variation on the Cross. Start with the Figure 8 Rope Turn. As the rope begins to cross from right to left, keep your left hand by your side while simultaneously crossing your right hand to the left. This will create the arc and allow you to jump through the opening. As the rope passes behind your head, uncross your hands and execute a 2 Foot Jump.

Double Matador

The Double Matador uses the exact same arm movements as the Matador, but this time when you enter the rope in the crossed position, you do a Double, or two rotations of the rope for each jump. Try to snap your wrists quickly so the rope rotates fast enough to complete the move.

Rump Jump

With both grips in one hand, swing the rope in a circular motion over your head, as if you're a cowboy ready to

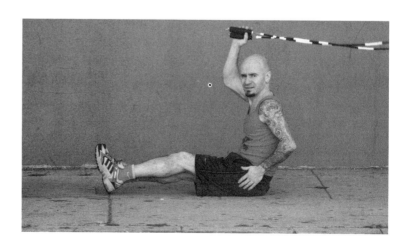

lasso a steer. Use your torso and opposite arm to help elevate your body as you bring the rope down to pass underneath your butt. Try one at a time and then a few consecutively. The Rump Jump guarantees that you'll be the life of the party and will have your audience howling with laughter.

Double Cross

The rope rotates twice for each time your feet hit the ground, as with a Double. On the first rotation of the rope, you execute a Cross. On the second rope rotation, the hands uncross. Double Crosses are a speed and power move that will have you sucking wind in no time at all. It's one continuous motion. It's

cross open / cross open / cross open / cross open / cross open / cross open / cross open / cross open.

Toe Catch Double Back

The Toe Catch Double Back is a modification of the Toe Catch and a great way to change direction of the rope. Start with a Figure 8. Execute a Toe Catch. Kick your leg forward, propelling the rope in a backward direction. Execute a Backward Double.

Underhand Pass Jump

The Underhand Pass Jump is a fancy handles-exchange move. With both handles in your right hand, you elevate and spread your legs apart with one leg forward and the other behind. Your right hand passes over your right leg, while your left arm reaches under your left leg and meets the right hand between your legs. Pass the handles from your right hand to your left.

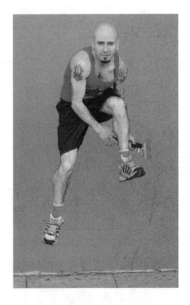

Backward Doubles

This jump is the same as Forward Doubles, but now you're executing the move with the rope rotating backward. Make sure to snap your wrists in small, tight circles.

Backward Double Cross

The Backward Double Cross is another jump that is exactly the same as the forward version, but with the rope rotating in the opposite direction. Remember to land softly and on the balls of your feet.

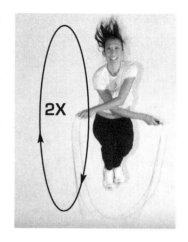

Running Doubles

Running Doubles are another high-end speed and power move. Start with a vertical Run. Whenever you're ready, execute a Double on one foot, alternating right and left, as you continue to move vertically.

Rope Release

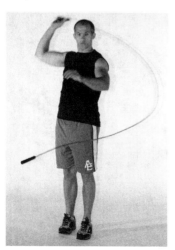

A cool-looking agility and finesse move. Begin with a Backward Figure 8 Rope Turn. As the rope comes forward, release both handles so the rope flies up and does two revolutions in the air before coming back to earth. Try to catch the rope smoothly as it comes down.

Triple Side Swing

With the Triple Side Swing, you execute a lightning-fast Figure 8 with your feet in the air, followed by a Figure 8 Entrance each time you elevate. It's

side side open / side side open / side side open /
side side open / side side open / side side open /
side side open / side side open.

Leg under Side Swing

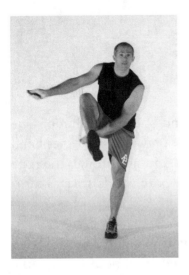

The Leg under Side Swing is a fancy rope turn. You step with one leg and kick the other leg up, swinging the rope over the kicking leg. The arms are essentially doing a Figure 8 with the hands separating and then coming together. If the right foot kicks up, the right arm swings to the outside of the leg and the left arm reaches slightly under the right leg. As the rope comes up and around, the right arm swings back over the right leg, flipping the rope around the extended leg. The hands meet together in front of the body to complete the Figure 8 as the right foot steps back down. Take two steps as you complete another Figure 8, and then try it again! Remember to practice on both your right and left sides. It's

kick swing step step / kick swing step step.

Leg under Arm Wrap

This fancy rope turn is an Arm Wrap including some legwork. If the rope is turning forward, step over the rope with your right leg and go directly into the Arm Wrap (the rope will still be under the lunging leg). Unwrap the rope, and when it's completely unwound, lift your foot up and transition into a Backward Figure 8. This move can be done forward or backward and on the right or left side. Go consecutively front and back or add some rope turns in between to create your own routines!

Leg under Side Swing Cross

This is a jump that starts the same way as the Leg under Side Swing. For this move, once your right leg kicks up, it stays up. The right arm then crosses over the right leg and

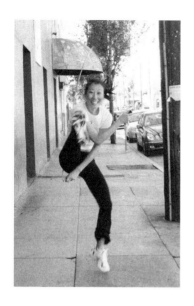

the left arm. The left arm remains slightly under the right leg, so your arms are now crossed. Jump over the rope with your left leg. As the rope comes up and over your head, uncross the rope and perform a Run onto the right leg, hopping over the rope for the final rotation of the jump. Finish it off with a regular 2 Foot Jump. It's

over cross uncross center / over cross uncross center.

Inverted Jump

Prepare with one Rope Turn and one 2 Foot Jump. One hand then crosses in front of the body and the other hand crosses behind the body, and you jump through the rope from the back angle. Make sure both hands are still turning the rope forward.

Inverted Doubles

Prepare and jump exactly as you would for the Inverted Jump. However, with the Double, you need to snap the wrist quickly to execute two rotations of the rope for every jump. So you cross one arm in front and one arm behind, then jump up while snapping your wrist for a Double jump.

Lateral Moves

Moving side to side with your rope is a fun way to add dynamics to your jumping. Whatever side you exit the rope, that's the direction you step out. That's the same side you start the Figure 8. If you exit to the right, the rope crosses over the body to complete the Figure 8. As the rope swings to the left, you step together with the other foot. Do a Half Figure 8 Entrance to jump through the rope and start the move again from the beginning.

It's slide together jump / slide together jump.

Part III

JUMP OUT
The RopeSport Way to a Healthier Lifestyle

Chapter 20

Alternative RopeSport Workouts

A unique thing about RopeSport is that with a little creativity you can design workouts for groups with specific needs or goals. This chapter will focus on alternative workouts for specific populations.

Kids' Workouts

About two years ago, working closely with the Los Angeles County Parks and Recreation Department, I started a program called RopeSport Nation and had the opportunity to teach hundreds of kids ages six to sixteen how to jump rope. The results were truly phenomenal. While my teaching experience may have played some part in the program's success, throwing out a bag of jump ropes and putting on some good music were just as important as anything else I did. The point is that kids *love* to jump rope, making the implementation of a successful jump rope program geared toward kids surprisingly simple.

Lazrael Lison, 25,
Personal trainer

Jumping rope is a kind of cardio you can't really get from any other exercise because you're working all your major muscle groups simultaneously, both upper and lower. It gets you in excellent physical condition and defines your muscles in a very short amount of time. You can burn a lot of calories. My clients like it because there are so many different jumps and moves that keep it exciting and motivating. I have clients as young as twenty-five and as old as seventy, and in very little time they have all the basic stuff down.

When I played college football a couple of years back, a lot of us jumped rope. That's why boxers are in such good shape—because they jump rope a lot. It is definitely great for footwork, agility, the whole nine yards.

There are an abundance of studies in recent years pointing to the fact that kids spend far too much time sitting in front of the television or computer and far too little time exercising. With the rates of childhood obesity and diabetes climbing at an alarming rate, both here and abroad, finding beneficial exercises that kids find fun and self-motivational couldn't be more important. Jumping rope is one of those exercises.

Here are a few options for implementing a successful jump rope program for kids.

Jump Rope Jam (35 to 40 minutes)

The Jump Rope Jam is loosely structured and allows participants of all skill levels and ages to participate. It is inclusive and easy to implement, making it ideally suited for K–12 physical education programs, Parks and Recreation Departments, YMCAs, and Boys & Girls Clubs. All you need to start are jump ropes, good music, and a group leader with basic jump rope proficiency.

- Preparation: Begin by making sure that all participants have a rope that is the proper length.
- Warm-up: A 10-minute warm-up consists of a few Basic Jumps and Resting Moves. During the warm-up there is a review of proper jumping technique and the introduction of one or two new jumps and moves each session so participants stay motivated.
- Stretching: The warm-up is followed by 5 minutes of upper- and lower-body stretches.
- Main Workout: For the main cardio portion of the jam session, put on some motivational music and allow participants to jump on their own for 15 to 20 minutes. Rotate around the room and give pointers to individual jumpers whenever necessary.
- Strength and Muscle Conditioning: After the jump cardio jam session, spend another 5 minutes doing some basic calisthenics that focus on different muscle groups. Include push-ups and sit-ups.
- Stretch: Finish with 5 minutes of upper- and lower-body stretches.

Jump Rope Games

Jump rope games are another great way to keep kids motivated. Here are a few examples of simple games and their skill levels that are easy to implement.

Maximum Number of Jumps in a Minute (Beginning) This can be done individually or as a team. One person jumps for one minute while another participant counts the number of jumps successfully completed. When done as a team, each member jumps for one minute and the team with the most total jumps is the winner.

Maximum Number of Consecutive Crosses (Intermediate/ Advanced) Who can do the most consecutive Crosses without missing? One person jumps while another one counts.

Maximum Number of Consecutive Doubles (Advanced)
Who can do the most consecutive Doubles without missing? One person jumps while another one counts.

Relay Races (Intermediate/Advanced) Split the participants into teams consisting of three or four members. Designate a start line and a finish line. One jumper from each team begins the race by doing a Run as fast as he or she can. When one jumper reaches the finish point, the next jumper from that team begins a Run. The first team to have all jumpers cross the finish line wins.

Run and Jump Cardio Blast (total workout time = 40 minutes)

The Run and Jump Cardio Blast is an outdoor workout that combines the best of two great cardio exercises, jumping rope and running. It's about getting back to the basics with a no-nonsense, fat-blasting cardio workout.

Warm-up

- Run (2 minutes): 30 percent of maximum

  Running Tip: Tie your jump rope around your waist, place it in a fanny pack, or just hold it in your hands during the Run portions of the workout. For increased difficulty, try running through the rope!

- Jump Rope (1 minute): Resting Moves (Figure 8s, 2 Turns to Each Side, or Step Touch)

Success Story

Steve Negri, 42, Financial consultant

I like RopeSport because it's low-impact and doesn't wear out my knees or my back. It keeps me toned and helps me maintain my weight. Jumping with other people keeps you motivated, and you feed off everybody's energy. You get the chance to show off a little with the different tricks and jumps.

Stretch

- Stretch (3 minutes): Include all the major muscle groups, upper and lower body.

Main Workout

- Jump Rope (1 minute): Resting Moves
- Run (2 minutes): 30 percent of maximum
- Jump Rope (2 minutes): Basic 2 Foot Jump
- Run (3 minutes): 50 percent of maximum
- Jump Rope (3 minutes): Basic Run (stationary or moving)
- Run (3 minutes): 70 percent of maximum
- Jump Rope (2 minutes): Basic 2 Foot Jump
- Jump Rope Interval (1 minute): Sprint Run (stationary)
- Run (3 minutes): 50 percent of maximum
- Jump Rope (2 minutes): Run (stationary or moving)
- Jump Rope Interval (1 minute): Sprint Run (stationary)

Cooldown

- Run (2 minutes): 30 percent of maximum
- Jump Rope (1 minute): Resting Moves

Strength and Muscle Conditioning

- Standing squats (1 minute)
- Lunges (1 minute)
- Push-ups (1 minute)
- Crunches (2 minutes)

Stretch

- Stretch (3 minutes): Include all the major muscle groups, upper and lower body.

**Circuit Jump Workout
(total workout time =
46 minutes)**

Read any leading fitness publication and you will see "circuit training" mentioned repeatedly as a proven, effective method of training. It combines strength and cardio in workout stations in which the participant does a specific exercise for 1 to 3 minutes before moving on to the next station (and exercise) with little or no break in between. I have been a strong proponent of circuit training for many years and believe it yields excellent results.

The following circuit jump workout combines jumping rope with calisthenics and can be done indoors or outdoors.

- Warm-up: Rope Turns with Resting Moves (5 minutes)
- Stretch: Upper- and Lower-Body Stretch (5 minutes)
- Jumping: 2 Foot Jump (1 minute)
- Strength: Standing Squats (1 minute)
- Jumping: Alternating Foot (2 minutes)
- Strength: Push-ups (1 minute)
- Jumping: Run (2 minutes)
- Strength: Lunges (2 minutes)
- Jumping: Rope Turns with Resting Moves (3 minutes)
- Strength: Abs (3 minutes)
- Jumping: Straddle Jump (1 minute)
- Strength: Squats (2 minutes)
- Jumping: Crosses (1 minute)
- Strength: Lunges (2 minutes)
- Jumping: Alternating Foot (3 minutes)
- Strength: Push-ups (1 minute)
- Jumping: Doubles or 2 Foot Jump (1 minute)
- Strength: Abs (2 minutes)
- Cooldown: Rope Turns with Resting Moves (3 minutes)
- Stretch: Upper- and Lower-Body Stretch (5 minutes)

Drills for Improving Athletic Skills

The following ten drills will improve speed and power development, agility, coordination, footwork, and timing. These same skills will lead to optimum performance in sports such as soccer, tennis, basketball, golf, football, ice hockey, volleyball, and baseball. The drills consist of moving vertically from a designated start to a finish point while the rope rotates forward or backward. I suggest a minimum of 25 meters from start to finish so you'll have sufficient space to repeat a move a number of times before you need to turn around. Before you begin these drills, take a moment to remind yourself of the importance of jumping with proper technique. Focus on landing softly.

Drill #1 (Basic)

Execute a Figure 8 Rope Turn (forward) while moving forward. When you reach your designated finish point, turn around and execute a Figure 8 Rope Turn (forward) while returning to your start point.

Drill #2 (Basic)

Execute a Figure 8 Rope Turn (backward) while moving forward to your designated finish point. Then turn around and execute a Figure 8 Rope Turn (backward) while you move forward and return to your start point.

Drill #3 (Basic)

Execute a Run (forward) while moving forward to your designated finish point. Then turn around and execute a Figure 8 Rope Turn (forward) while returning to your start point.

Drill #4 (Intermediate)

Execute a Knee Up Run (forward) while moving forward to your designated finish point. Then turn around and execute a Knee Up Run (forward) while returning to your start point.

Drill #5 (Intermediate)

Execute a Slalom (forward) while moving forward to your designated finish point. Then turn around and execute a Slalom (forward) while returning to your start point.

Drill #6 (Intermediate)

Execute a Run (backward) while moving forward to your designated finish point. Then turn around and execute a Run (backward) while moving forward, returning to your start point.

Drill #7 (Advanced)

Execute Running Crosses (forward) while moving forward to your designated finish point. Then stay facing the same direction and execute Running Crosses (forward) while moving backward, returning to your start point.

Drill #8 (Advanced)

Execute Doubles (forward) while moving forward to your designated finish point. Then turn around and execute a Run (forward) while returning to your start point.

Drill #9 (Advanced)

Execute Doubles (forward) while moving forward to your designated finish point. Then turn around and execute Doubles (forward) while returning to your start point.

Drill #10 (Advanced)

Execute 2 Foot Jump (backward) while moving backward to your designated finish point. Then turn around and execute a 2 Foot Jump (backward) while moving backward, returning to your start point.

Chapter 21

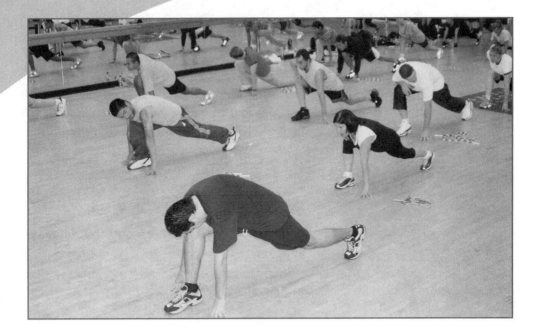

Stretching

The importance of stretching on a regular basis cannot be emphasized enough. It is a critical component in keeping your muscles healthy and minimizing any chance of injury. The key to becoming more flexible is to stretch on a regular basis, each and every day if possible.

Stretch each individual muscle group for 20 to 60 seconds. It's a natural reflex for your muscles to tighten up during the first few seconds that you try to stretch them—it is the body's way of protecting against injury—so be sure to hold the stretch long enough to allow the muscle to relax. If and when the muscle feels ready, you can *slowly* go a little deeper into the stretch.

Proper breathing plays a central role in keeping the muscles relaxed. Try to direct your breath right into the specific muscle group you're stretching. *If* you feel comfortable, try to go a little deeper into the stretch with each exhale.

It's just as important to stretch at the end of your workout as at the beginning—in some ways more so. First, it will allow you to bring your heart rate down slowly and safely. Second, you can achieve maximum flexibility because your muscles are warm after you've jumped. Finally, after completing an intense workout during which your adrenaline has been pumping, it feels good to relax with a proper stretch before you return to the real world with all that it brings.

While there are literally hundreds of effective stretches, here are some of my favorites.

Neck

Head Rotation   Begin by slowly turning your head from right to left and then left to right. Keep your head upright as it turns 180 degrees from shoulder to shoulder. Continue to repeat.

Head Rolls   Roll your head forward and down in a semicircle from one side to the other with your chin tucked in. Continue to repeat.

Note: *Do not* let your head drop back behind you, something that can easily result in a bad muscle pull to your neck.

Deltoids (Shoulders)

Shoulder Circles   Circle both shoulders forward in small, controlled movements. Keep your neck long and relaxed. Continue to repeat.

Circle both shoulders backward at the same time. Continue to repeat.

Alternating Shoulder Circles   Circle your right shoulder forward one time. Then circle your left shoulder forward one time. Continue to repeat, alternating right and left.

Circle your right shoulder backward one time. Then circle your left shoulder backward one time. Continue to repeat, alternating right and left.

Triceps (Back of Arm)

Arms across the Body   Bring your right arm in front of you and across your body. Use your left arm to grasp your right arm near your elbow. Gently pull with your left hand to maximize the stretch.

Repeat the stretch with your left arm positioned in front.

Arms Cocked behind Head   Position your right arm behind your head with your elbow bent and pointing up. Use your left hand to grasp your right arm near your elbow. Gently pull toward the left with your left hand to maximize the stretch.

Repeat the stretch with your left arm positioned behind your head.

Oblique (Side Abdominal)

Waist Bend   Place your feet shoulder-width apart. Place your left hand on your left hip. Bend over from your waist sideways and to your left with your right hand reaching over your head. Extend as far as you can comfortably go as you try to keep a good line and isolate the stretch to your side.

Repeat with your right hand placed on your right hip, bending to your right with your left hand reaching out.

Erector Spinae (Lower Back)

Flex and Extend   With your legs shoulder-width apart, bend forward at the waist and position your hands on or just above your knees. Start by contracting your stomach so your back is flexed and curls upward. After holding this position briefly, release and press down into your lower back so it is arched for maximum extension. This is also known as the supported cat stretch. Continue to repeat.

Pectorals (Chest) and Biceps

Arms Clasped behind the Back   Clasp your hands behind your back. Try to straighten your arms while you slowly raise them upward so you feel the stretch in your chest and biceps.

Figure 8   With both grips in one hand, execute a very slow Figure 8 Rope Turn (one hand). For maximum effect, exaggerate the crossing motion. Switch the grips to your other hand and repeat the movement.

Gluteals and Abductors (Butt and Hips)

Hip Circles   Stand with your feet shoulder-width apart. Circle your hips clockwise a few times. Then rotate them counterclockwise a few times. Keep it nice and slow.

Quadriceps (Front of Thighs)

Standing Quadriceps Stretch   Stand on your right leg only with your left leg behind you and bent at the knee. Use your left hand to grasp your left foot. Pull slowly with your left hand until you feel the stretch in your left quadricep. If you're having trouble balancing on one leg, extend your right arm out to help steady you. If a wall or a chair is nearby, feel free to put your right hand against it to keep your balance.
Repeat the stretch standing on your left leg.

Groin

Runner's Stretch   Position your left leg in front of you with your left knee bent. Make sure your left knee does not extend past your left toe. Your right leg is positioned behind you and remains straight but not rigid. You should feel the stretch in your groin area. Be careful to only go down as far as you're comfortable. This stretch can feel awkward, so focus on doing it slowly and safely.

Repeat on the other side with your right leg bent in front and your left leg behind.

Hamstrings (Back of Thigh)

Standing Stretch   Bend at the waist and extend your right leg forward and away from your body with your right heel digging into the ground. Your right leg should be straight but not rigid. Use your right hand to grasp your right toe. At the same time, your left leg is bent with your left hand placed on your left hip. Most of your weight is on your left leg. As you bend forward you should feel the stretch in the back of your right thigh (your hamstring muscle). If you want to increase the stretch, try to flatten your lower back. Keep it nice and slow and gentle. Breathe right into the muscle.

Repeat the stretch with your left leg forward and your right leg behind.

Gastrocnemius, Soleus, and Tibialis Anterior (Calf and Shins)

Roll Front and Back   Stand with slightly bent knees and your feet shoulder-width apart. With your hands placed on your hips, roll forward and up on the balls of your feet so you feel the stretch in your calves. Then shift your weight so you roll back on your heels with your toes in the air. You should feel the stretch in your shins. Continue to repeat.

Calf Stretch   Stand with your feet spread apart in a mini-Lunge. Place both hands on the leg that is positioned in front and lean forward slightly. Feel the stretch in the calf of your back leg. Reverse the position of your feet and repeat.

Ankles and Tibialis Anterior (Shins)

Ankle Circles   Stand on your right foot only. Circle your left foot clockwise a few times, then counterclockwise a few times. Keep the movement tight and controlled.

Repeat while standing on your left foot only with your right foot circling in both directions.

Tibialis Anterior (Shins)

Toe Taps (up and down; in and out)   Stand with your feet shoulder-width apart and your right foot slightly in front. With your right knee bent slightly, tap your right toe. Bring it up as high as you can while tapping it. This will help to stretch and warm up your shins, a muscle group that's often overlooked but that's very important to focus on when you're doing any impact exercise, including jumping rope. Continue tapping up and down, but rotate your foot in and out (right and left) simultaneously. The full range of motion should be about 90 degrees. Repeat the sequence with your left foot tapping up and down, then in and out.

Glutes (Butt) and Lower Back

Supine Knee to Chest   Lie on your back with your head and neck relaxed. Bring your right knee into your chest. Clasp your hands near your right knee and slowly pull. You should feel the stretch in your lower back. Repeat on the other side.

Twist to Side   Lie on your back and pull your right knee in to your chest. Place your left hand on top of your right knee. Twist over onto your left side. Keep your shoulders on the ground so you get a good stretch through your lower back. Repeat on the other side.

Hamstrings, Groin, Calves, Hips, and Sides

Seated Butterfly   While seated, bring the soles of your feet together so they're touching. Grasp your feet with your hands. Let your knees gently open to the sides. Slowly lean your body forward as far as is comfortable. Feel the stretch in your groin area and hips.

Jonathon Burdeos, 47, Accounting

I always feel great after jumping. I come from a family with a history of heart disease, so it's especially important for me to stay in good shape. You get a good tone and a good burn. I love jumping to music. The basic techniques are very easy to learn.

Seated Legs Extended In a seated position, straighten your legs in front of you. Extend your body forward and reach toward your toes. Keep your head and shoulders relaxed. While you hold the position, point and flex your toes to increase the stretch in your calves and hamstrings.

Seated Straddle Spread your legs out in front of you in a straddle or V position as far as you're comfortable. Lean over to your left side with your right arm over your head. As you hold the position you should feel the stretch in your right side and hamstring. Slowly bring yourself back to center position and lean over to your right with your left hand over your head. Come back to center.

Slowly extend your torso and reach forward so your torso is between your legs. Feel the stretch in your hamstrings, hips, and groin.

Deep Breathing I always like to finish the stretch by taking a few deep breaths. Fill your lungs with air. Feel each individual breath entering and leaving your body. Center yourself.

Chapter 22

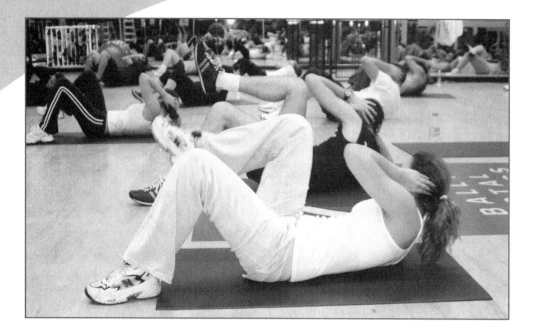

Strength Training, Muscle Toning, and Shaping

There is general agreement among fitness experts that combining cardio and strength training is the most effective way to work out and will result in maximum benefits. That's why I almost always spend a minimum of a few minutes doing a variety of strength-oriented exercises after I've finished jumping. Strength training also burns a lot of fat, so if you're trying to lose weight, you should consider it an essential part of your workout.

Finally, if you're like a vast majority of people who want to develop shapely defined muscles from head to toe, you've got to strength-train.

The breathing technique for these strength-training exercises is to exhale while the muscle you're working is contracting and fully engaged, and to inhale as you release the contraction. For example, when you're doing a push-up, exhale as you push up and inhale on the way down.

I suggest that you alternate pace when doing many of these exercises. A majority of the time, do slow, controlled repetitions. This forces you to focus on the muscle group you're working, rather than using momentum to complete the movement. Using faster double-time pulses is an effective training technique to sculpt and define a particular muscle group.

Quadriceps, Hamstrings, and Glutes

Squats

Begin with your knees slightly bent and shoulder-width apart. Keeping your chest lifted, slowly lower yourself as far as is comfortable, but *do not* let your butt drop lower than your knees or a 90-degree angle. Use your quadriceps, hamstrings, and glutes to bring yourself up slowly until you're back to your starting position, standing with slightly bent knees. Try to keep the movement slow and controlled. Within just a few repetitions you should feel it working the upper part of your legs and butt.

You can modify Standing Squats to include Squats with Knee Lifts, Squats with Side Leg Raises, Squats with Back Leg Lifts, Squats with Hamstring Curls, Plié Squats, and Squats of double speed with a smaller range of motion. I would recommend that you alternate Standing Squats with these variations to keep your workout motivational and challenging. These variations also work the muscle from different angles, a strength-training technique that is very beneficial.

Lunges

Alternating Lunges are one of the best exercises you can do for your butt and thighs, and they're among my personal favorites. Start in a standing position. *Slowly* take a step forward with your right leg and lower your body toward the ground with your left leg positioned behind you. Continue to lower yourself as far as you can comfortably go. As you lower yourself, make sure that your right knee never extends past your right foot, avoiding unnecessary strain on your knee. After you reach the lowest comfortable position, slowly raise yourself up and step back with your right leg so you're standing again. Remember to keep the movement slow and controlled. Repeat the same movement with your left leg lunging forward and your right leg positioned behind you.

You can vary Alternating Lunges with Same-Leg Lunges and Walking Lunges (where you move forward while executing Alternating Lunges).

If you do a few minutes of Lunges with each workout, you should have no trouble developing a nice, shapely butt.

Back, Chest, Biceps, Triceps, and Shoulders

Push-ups

I suggest doing a few sets of push-ups toward the end of your workout. They are an excellent overall toning exercise for all the major muscle groups of your upper body. Feel free to do them on your knees, a modification that's a little easier. Your abdominals should be tight throughout the entire movement so your back is supported. Be sure not to arch your back. As you push up and straighten your arms, try not to lock your elbows.

Tricep Dips

Tricep Dips focus on the backs of your arms. In a seated position, your legs are bent in front of your body with the feet placed flat on the ground. Your hands should be placed hip-width apart below your shoulders. Balance on your heels as you slowly raise yourself up and down for a killer triceps workout.

Abdominals

Here are a few of the many effective exercises you can do for your stomach. Regardless of which abdominal exercises you choose, make sure you do the entire movement slowly and carefully in order to protect your lower back and neck.

Crunches

Lie down on the floor with your hands placed behind your head. Your feet are flat on the ground and your knees are bent. Start with your shoulders off the ground and your elbows out. Your lower back remains pressed into the ground. As you exhale, contract your stomach while raising your shoulders and chin to the highest point you're comfortable with. Your abdominals should be doing all the work, so try not to pull on your neck as you raise up. Hold at the highest point, or the peak of the movement, for a split second. Inhale while you slowly lower until you reach where you started. Continue to repeat.

Rotation Crunches

You begin Alternating Rotation Crunches in the exact same position as you do with regular Crunches. Your hands are placed behind your head. Your shoulders are off the ground and your elbows are out. Your lower back remains pressed into the ground. However, instead of lifting straight up as you contract your abdominal muscles, you twist your right shoulder over to the left side of your body as far as you can comfortably go. After holding to the twist for a split second, you untwist as you lower yourself back to the ground to where you started. Repeat the same movement on the other side with your left shoulder twisting over to your right side. Continue to repeat.

The primary muscles you're working with Rotation Crunches are your obliques or the side of your stomach, affectionately known as your love handles.

Knee/Elbow Crunches

Knee/Elbow crunches are excellent for working your lower abdominals. Start in the same position as you do for regular and Alternating Rotation Crunches. Bring your feet off the ground and your elbows in at the same time until they touch. With your elbows and knees touching, hold the contraction for a split second. Release the contraction and slowly lower yourself to the ground. Be careful not to pull on your neck with this exercise. Continue to repeat.

Chapter 23

RopeSport for Fitness Professionals

Group exercise instructors, personal trainers, and physical education teachers can all benefit from teaching RopeSport. Due to the modifications that are an integral part of the teaching method, effective and motivational workouts can be specifically designed for group classes at gyms, individual clients, or K–12 students. A wide variety of ages and skill levels can be accommodated. Cost is also not a significant factor—for less than the price of a single treadmill you can equip an entire gym or school with a lot of jump ropes. RopeSport classes are often composed equally of men and women, something that makes it rare in group exercise environments, where getting men to participate has always been a struggle. That is a concrete, positive selling point for potential male members and something that keeps the management team happy. Little boys like to jump just as much as little girls, making Rope-Sport ideally suited for physical education programs in schools.

It's pretty easy to implement a successful jump rope program. All you need are good-quality jump ropes and an instructor with basic jump rope proficiency. So you don't need to know more than a handful of jumps and tricks to get started—as with most other disciplines, *what's most important is how good a teacher you are.*

What qualities make for a good jump rope instructor? At the very top of the list is having a thorough knowledge of safety considerations in working with a wide variety of people—old, young, in good shape or not. Any good instructor also has the knowledge and the ability to demonstrate the *modifications* in order to teach people of various skill levels how to benefit from their very first workout. You also need to be able to clearly demonstrate proper jumping technique for any moves you're teaching. Further, a quality instructor needs to be able to watch someone jump and quickly analyze their technique, including the ability to gently make corrections when necessary. You also need to help your clients and students understand that missing is an integral part of jumping. Another thing that makes for a good jump rope instructor is bringing positive energy and patience to each and every workout. And finally, you've got to make it *fun*.

If you can effectively demonstrate and impart this knowledge, I guarantee that whoever you're teaching will be eternally grateful to you for introducing them to jumping rope the RopeSport way.

Chapter 24

Effective Training and a Healthy Lifestyle

Rest between Workouts

You've got to make sure you get enough sleep and rest between workouts. I suggest taking at least two days off a week to give your body time to recover and your muscles a chance to heal and recuperate. If you're training intelligently and eating properly, working out five days a week is more than enough. Overtraining is a real problem for many people who become obsessed with working out for a variety of unhealthy reasons and should be avoided. There have been times over the twenty-plus years that I've been working out when I have been guilty of overtraining. I can tell you from firsthand experience that you don't need to walk around feeling tired all the time to achieve the results you're looking for. In fact, proper rest will give you the energy you need to train intensely, while at the same time minimizing any chance of injuries that often occur because you're overly tired and your muscles have not had time to recover between workouts. In addition to weekly rest days, it's also a good idea to take two weeks off a year when you do no training whatsoever. For example, take a full week off in the fall and another week off in the spring. These week-long breaks will give your body a chance to completely heal and rejuvenate itself. Don't be surprised if you come back to your workouts stronger than ever, both physically and mentally!

Meditation and Jump Rope Zen

In the past few years meditation has become an important part of my life, and I highly recommend it. In today's fast-paced world it seems as if we're cramming more and more into our waking hours. As president of RopeSport I needed to take care of a multitude of daily tasks and responsibilities at the same time I was writing this book, forcing me to work long hours for many months. One of the ways I was able to cope with this workload and the resultant pressure was through a disciplined meditation practice. It's my firm belief that finding some stillness each and every day is as important as anything else in your life, including exercise. I also believe that meditation improves your ability to concentrate, something that will have a positive affect on your jumping. While you need to concentrate when you jump, you need to stay loose and relaxed at the same time. I sometimes refer to this feeling of relaxed concentration as "jump rope zen."

Mixing Up Your Cardio Workouts

In addition to jumping rope, I strongly encourage you to mix up your training by periodically doing other cardio workouts, including step aerobics, kickboxing, and spinning. All of these are beneficial in different ways, and varying your workouts helps you stay motivated over the long haul. The truth is that there are many different exercises that can work, and anyone who tells you that their way is the only way is—in my opinion—an egomaniac or an ignoramus. That being said, it's only natural to gravitate toward the exercises that you find most motivational, and I am supremely confident that you will see for yourself that jumping rope is one of the most beneficial and fun cardio workouts in existence. It's been my experience that after you start jumping rope the RopeSport way, you'll spend a lot less time doing other cardio workouts.

Combining Jumping Rope with Weight Lifting

Throughout the many years I've been teaching jumping rope I've had the opportunity to work closely with many highly respected authorities, including strength and conditioning experts, coaches, athletes, physicians, and fitness professionals. The overwhelming consensus among these experts is that combining cardio and strength training is the most effective and beneficial way to train. That's why I strongly recommend weight lifting as the ideal complement to your RopeSport workouts, ensuring that you are getting the best possible results in the least amount of time.

Duration and Frequency of Workout

How frequently and how long you should jump for depends on a number of variables, including your age, your level of physical conditioning, how intensely you're training, and whether you're doing Resting Moves most of the time or jumping through the rope for most of your workout.

As a general rule, I suggest that beginners start jumping two or three times a week for approximately 20 minutes per workout. As your jumping skills and stamina improve, try increasing to three or four times a week for 30 to 45 minutes per workout. If you're an advanced jumper and really trying to push yourself, you can jump four to five times a week for as long as 45 to 60 minutes per workout.

Success Story

Phil Gibson, 59, Retired firefighter

I like to jump rope because it's challenging and fun. Just by turning the rope you burn a lot of calories. RopeSport can be for any age group. With the different modifications and Resting Moves, everybody can work at their own level.

Photo Credits

Index

abdominals
  strength training for,
    215–216
  stretches for, 207–208
abductors, stretches for, 208
active rest, 5
Advanced Jumps, 146–151
  Alternating High Kicks,
    147
  Can Can, 147–148
  combinations, 153–171
  Cross variations, 151
  Heel Click, 148
  Knee Up Cross Over, 150
  Running Man, 148–149
  Touch Front and Back,
    149–150
  Triples, 150–151
  vertical movement,
    151–152
Advanced RopeSport Work-
    outs, 172–188
  grid, 187–188
  Workout 1, 172–176
  Workout 2, 176–180

Workout 3, 180–183
  Workout 4, 183–187
Alternating Foot (Figure 8
    Bouncing), 47, 50, 56–58,
    78–79
Alternating High Kicks, 147
Alternating Knee Up, 79–80
Alternating Lunges, 214
Alternative RopeSport work-
    outs, 197–204
ankles, stretches for, 210
apparel, 29
arms
  strength training for,
    214–216
  stretches for, 207, 208
Arm Wrap, 65–66, 68

back
  strength training for,
    214–215
  stretches for, 208, 210
Backward Double Cross,
    192
Backward Doubles, 192

Backward Figure 8 Entrance, 114–115
Backward 2 Foot Jump, 80–81
backward variations of jumps, 64, 115. *See also individual names of jumps*
Basic Jumps, 73–82
  Alternating Foot, 78–79
  Alternating Knee Up, 79–80
  Backward 2 Foot Jump, 80–81
  Boxer Shuffle, 77–78
  combinations, 83–95
  Cross, 81–82
  Front/Back, 74
  Lunge (Scissor), 75–76
  Run, 76
  Slalom, 74
  Straddle, 75
  Toe In/Toe Out, 77
Basic RopeSport Workouts, 96–106
  grid, 106
  Workout 1, 96–98
  Workout 2, 99–101
  Workout 3, 101–103
  Workout 4, 103–105
Basic Rope Turns, 62–64
Behind the Back, 67
biceps
  strength training for, 214–215
  stretches for, 208
Body Wrap, 67
Boxer Shuffle, 50, 77–78
breathing, 31–32, 206, 213
Bunny Hop, 35, 61
butt, stretches for, 208, 210
Butterfly, 67

calories, 11
calves, stretches for, 209, 210–211
Can Can, 147–148
cardiovascular portion of workout, 48–53
  strength training and, 212
  variety in, 221–222
chest
  strength training for, 214–215
  stretches for, 208
children, 6, 15, 22, 197–204
circuit jump workout, 202
clothing, 29
cool down, 53
Cross, 81–82
Cross variations, 151
Crunches, 215–216

deltoids, stretches for, 207
Double Bounce, 112–113
Double Cross, 191
Double Dutch style, 17
Double Matador, 190
Doubles, 115
drills for improving athletic skills, 203–204

equipment, 13–14, 25–32
erector spinae, stretches for, 208
Extreme Jumps, 189–194
  Backward Double Cross, 192
  Backward Doubles, 192
  Double Cross, 191
  Double Matador, 190
  Inverted Doubles, 194
  Inverted Jump, 194
  lateral moves, 194

Leg under Arm Wrap, 193
Leg under Side Swing, 193
Leg under Side Swing
    Cross, 193–194
Matador, 190
Rope Release, 192
Rump Jump, 190–191
Running Doubles, 192
Toe Catch Double Back,
    191
Triple Side Swing, 193
Underhand Pass Jump,
    191

fat burning, 11, 46
Figure 8, 55–56
    Backward Figure 8
        Entrance, 114–115
    Bouncing (Alternating
        Foot), 47, 50, 56–58,
        78–79
    Entrance, 58
    Exit, 61
    High and Low, 64
fitness level requirements,
    21–22
fitness professionals, Rope-
    Sport for, 217–219
flexibility, 54
Foot Cross, 111–112
FreeStyle jumping, 52–53
FreeStyle Rope Turns, 41–42,
    47, 49
FreeStyle soloing, 43–44
Front/Back, 74
fundamentals, 55–61
Funky Step Touch, 65

games, jump rope, 199–200
gastrocnemius, stretches for,
    209

gluteals
    strength training for,
        213–214
    stretches for, 208, 210
going in/out of the rope,
    42–43
groin, stretches for, 209,
    210–211

hair, 29
Half Figure 8 Entrance, 114
hamstrings
    strength training for,
        213–214
    stretches for, 209, 210–211
handle design, 26, 38
Hand over Hand, 66
Heel Back, 110–111
Heel Catch, 68–69
Heel Click, 148
Heel Together, 111
High Knee Run, 108–109
hips, stretches for, 208,
    210–211
history, of jumping rope,
    16–17
Holding Cross, 112
hydration, 31. See also work-
    out format

impact, 22
instructors, RopeSport for,
    217–219
Intermediate Jumps, 107–115
    Backward Figure 8
        Entrance, 114–115
    Backward variations, 115
    combinations, 116–133
    Double Bounce, 112–113
    Doubles, 115
    Foot Cross, 111–112

Intermediate Jumps
  (continued)
  Half Figure 8 Entrance, 114
  Heel Back, 110–111
  Heel Together, 111
  High Knee Run, 108–109
  Holding Cross, 112
  Side to Side, 109
  Sprint Intervals, 113–114
  Step Kick Back, 110
  Step Kick Forward, 109,
    110
  Toe Heel, 112
  The Twist, 107–108
  V Jump, 108
Intermediate RopeSport
  Workouts, 134–145
  grid, 145
  Workout 1, 134–137
  Workout 2, 137–139
  Workout 3, 139–142
  Workout 4, 142–145
Intermediate Rope Turns,
  64–66
interval training, 5
Inverted Doubles, 194
Inverted Jump, 194

jump combinations, 51–52
  Advanced, 153–171
  Basic, 83–95
  Intermediate, 116–133
jumping mats, 30
jump rope games, 199–200
Jump Rope Jam, 198–199
"jump rope zen," 221

Knee/Elbow Crunches, 216
Knee Up Cross Over, 150

lateral moves, 194

leather ropes, 27
legs
  strength training for,
    213–214, 216
  stretches for, 208, 209,
    210
Leg under Arm Wrap, 193
Leg under Side Swing, 193
Leg under Side Swing Cross,
  193–194
length of ropes, 28–29
lifestyle, 220–222
locations for jumping rope,
  18–19, 23
Long Jump, 52
Los Angeles County Parks
  and Recreation Depart-
  ment, 197
lower back, stretches for,
  208, 210
Lunges, 75–76
  Alternating, 214
  Funky Step Touch, 65
  Same-Leg, 214
  Walking, 214

Matador, 190
mats, 30
meditation, 221
"missing," 40
modifications, 5, 31
motivation, 22–23
muscle conditioning, 53–54,
  212–216. See also individual names of muscles
music, 29–30

neck, stretches for, 206–207

obliques, stretches for,
  207–208

One-Hand Variation, 64
overtraining, 220–222

pectorals, stretches for, 208
philosophy of RopeSport,
     41–44
physiology, 19–20
plastic-beaded ropes, 27
practice, importance of, 8

quadriceps
  strength training for,
     213–214
  stretches for, 208

Recovery, 36–38, 50
Recovery Jumps, 51
resistance, 20
rest, training and, 220–222
Resting Moves, 36–38, 50,
     62–64
  backward, 64
  Figure 8, 55–56
Rope Release, 192
RopeSport LLC, 3–4
  accessibility of, 6–7, 14–15
  for children, 6, 15, 22,
     197–204
  fitness level requirements,
     21–22
  for fitness professionals,
     217–219
  fundamentals, 55–61
  for instructors, 217–219
  philosophy of, 41–44
  RopeSport Nation, 197
  safety, 30–31, 45–46
Rope Turns, 62–69
  backward, 64
  Basic, Resting Moves,
     62–64

Figure 8, 55–56
  Intermediate, 64–66
Rotation Crunches, 216
Rump Jump, 190–191
Run, 50, 76
Run and Jump Cardio Blast,
     200–201
Running Doubles, 192
Running Man, 148–149

safety, 30–31, 45–46
Same-Leg Lunges, 214
Scissor (Lunge), 75–76
segmented ropes, 27
shins, stretches for, 209, 210
shoulders
  strength training for,
     214–215
  stretches for, 207
side abdominals, stretches
     for, 207–208
sides, stretches for, 210–211
Side to Side, 109
Single-Rope Jumping style,
     17–18
Slalom, 74
sleep, 220
soleus, stretches for, 209
speed ropes, 27
Sprint Intervals, 50–51,
     113–114
squats, 213
Step Kick Back, 110
Step Kick Forward, 109, 110
Straddle, 75
strength training, 53–54,
     212–216, 222. *See also*
     *individual names of mus-
     cles*
stretching, 45, 48, 54,
     205–211

teams, 19
technique, 33–35
 instruction on, 217–219
 proper form checklist,
   35–36
 Resting Moves and Recov-
   ery, 36–38
 Three-Step Breakdown,
   38–40
thighs, stretches for, 208, 209
Three-Step Breakdown,
   38–40
3 Turns to Each Side, 66–67
Through the Legs, 68
tibialis anterior, stretches for,
   209, 210
time, for workout, 23–24
Toe Catch Double Back, 191
Toe Catch with a Kick, 69
Toe Heel, 112
Toe In/Toe Out, 77
toning, 12, 53–54, 212–216.
   See also individual names
   of muscles
Touch Front and Back,
   149–150
training, 12, 13, 33–40,
   220–222
triceps
 strength training for,
   214–215
 stretches for, 207
Triples, 150–151
Triple Side Swing, 193
true arc, 26
The Twist, 107–108

2 Foot Jump, 50, 59–61
2 Turns Step Touch, 63–64
2 Turns to Each Side, 47,
   62–63

Underhand Pass Jump, 191
Under the Leg Pass, 68
United States Amateur Jump
   Rope Federation, 19

vertical movement, 151–152
V Jump, 108

Walking Lunges, 214
warm-up, 46–48
water, 31. *See also* workout
   format
weighted ropes, 28
weight lifting, 222
Winkler, Martin, 1–2
workout format
 cardio portion, 48–53
 cool down, 53
 duration, frequency of, 222
 healthy lifestyle and,
   220–222
 muscle conditioning, toning, 53–54
 safety, 45–46
 warm-up, 46–48
 See also Advanced Rope-
   Sport Workouts; Alternative RopeSport Workouts;
   Basic RopeSport Work-
   outs; Intermediate Rope-
   Sport Workouts